Navigating Mental Health in the Digital Age

How Technology, Social Media, and Digital Overload Impact Our Minds and Well-Being

Table of Contents

Introduction 1

Chapter 1 The Age of Digital Dependency 4

    The Rise of Social Media and Its Influence 5

    Smartphones: A Double-Edged Sword for Mental Health 7

    The Addiction to Screen Time and Its Consequences 9

Chapter 2 The Mental Health Crisis: A Global Perspective 12

    Increased Anxiety and Depression Among Youth 13

    Social Media's Role in Escalating Mental Health Issues............15

    Global Studies: What the Data Reveals......................................18

Chapter 3 The Illusion of Connection 21

    Superficial Interactions: How Social Media Alters Relationships 22

    The Impact of "Likes" and Validation on Self-Esteem 24

    The Anxiety of Missing Out: FOMO and Its Effects 27

Chapter 4 Cyberbullying and Online Harassment 30

    The Prevalence of Cyberbullying in the Digital World..............31

Psychological Consequences of Online Abuse 33

Strategies for Combating Cyberbullying 36

Chapter 5 The Role of Digital Detox in Mental Health 39

Why Unplugging is Essential for Mental Wellness 40

How to Start a Digital Detox: Practical Tips 42

The Long-Term Benefits of Reduced Screen Time 44

Chapter 6 The Effects of Constant Information Overload. 47

The 24/7 News Cycle and Its Psychological Toll 48

Navigating the Stress of Digital Information Consumption 50

Finding Balance: Curating Your Digital Environment 53

Chapter 7 Mindfulness in the Digital Age 56

What Is Digital Mindfulness? 57

How Mindfulness Can Help Mitigate Digital Stress 58

Tools and Techniques for Practicing Mindfulness Online 61

Chapter 8 The Impact of Social Comparison on Mental Health 64

The "Highlight Reel" Culture of Social Media 65

How Comparison Affects Our Self-Worth 67

Breaking the Cycle: Strategies for Healthy Self-Perception 69

Chapter 9 The Digital Divide: Mental Health in the Age of Inequality 73

Access to Technology and Mental Health Disparities................74

How Socioeconomic Status Affects Digital Wellness 76

Bridging the Gap: Solutions for Mental Health Equity..............79

Chapter 10 Children, Teens, and Screen Time 82

The Impact of Social Media on Adolescent Development.........83

Parental Control and Setting Boundaries 86

Teaching Kids Healthy Digital Habits 88

Chapter 11 Digital Addiction: Causes, Consequences, and Solutions..91

Why Technology is Addictive..92

The Psychological and Physical Toll of Digital Addiction 95

Treatment Approaches for Digital Dependency........................97

Chapter 12 Digital Addiction: Causes, Consequences, and Solutions..100

Setting Boundaries: The Role of Self-Regulation 101

How to Design a Mindful Digital Routine 104

Building a Supportive Digital Community...............................106

Introduction

In just a few short decades, technology has transformed the way we live, work, and interact. What was once considered a luxury or novelty has evolved into an essential part of daily life. The internet, smartphones, social media, and endless digital platforms have seamlessly woven themselves into the fabric of our existence. We can now connect with friends, shop, work, and access information all at the tap of a finger. The shift from traditional forms of communication to digital communication has not only affected the way we interact with others but has also shaped our values, perceptions, and habits. Technology has infiltrated almost every facet of our lives, becoming a necessary tool for both personal and professional success. However, this digital shift comes with its own set of challenges, particularly when it comes to our mental health and well-being.

The pervasive presence of technology has resulted in a new phenomenon—constant connectivity. We are perpetually plugged in, checking emails, social media notifications, and news updates. While this constant flow of information can seem exciting and efficient, it takes a toll on our mental health. The psychological effects of living in a hyper-connected world are profound. Studies show that constant screen time and exposure to digital content can lead to feelings of anxiety, stress, and depression. The pressure to maintain an online persona, the addiction to instant gratification, and the exposure to harmful content can erode our sense of self-worth and emotional stability.

This constant connection often results in information overload, where the brain is bombarded with more data than it can process. The consequences are severe—difficulty focusing, decision fatigue, and a sense of being overwhelmed. Moreover, the digital world is often curated to show the best sides of people's lives, which leads to unhealthy comparisons and self-esteem issues. Social media platforms, with their emphasis on "likes" and validation, have created a cycle of dependence that has deeply impacted how we value ourselves and others. As we spend more time online, we risk becoming disconnected from the real world, losing touch with our emotions and genuine human connections.

As we become more reliant on technology, the need for digital well-being has never been more urgent. Digital well-being refers to the practices, strategies, and tools that allow individuals to maintain a healthy balance between their digital and offline lives. It involves setting boundaries, practicing mindfulness, and creating an intentional relationship with technology. Digital well-being is about taking control of how and when we use technology, ensuring that it serves us rather than dictates our lives.

The growing concern over digital addiction and its effects on mental health has led to an increasing number of people seeking ways to reclaim their time and focus. From setting screen time limits to engaging in regular digital detoxes, individuals are exploring strategies to combat the negative effects of technology. It is becoming clear that we must learn how to live in harmony with technology rather than allowing it to dominate our lives. By understanding the psychological impact of constant connectivity and adopting strategies for digital well-being, we can pave the way for a healthier, more balanced relationship with the digital world.

This book aims to explore the intricate relationship between technology and mental health, shedding light on the challenges and providing actionable steps to improve digital well-being. Through this journey, we will better understand how we can navigate the digital age while prioritizing our mental and emotional health.

Chapter 1
The Age of Digital Dependency

In today's world, digital dependency has become a defining characteristic of modern life. The rapid rise of social media, smartphones, and constant internet access has made it nearly impossible to go a day without interacting with some form of technology. What started as a tool to enhance communication and streamline tasks has evolved into an essential part of our daily existence. People of all ages are increasingly tethered to their devices, whether for work, socializing, or entertainment. This constant connection has fundamentally shifted the way we interact with the world, creating both opportunities and challenges. While technology offers numerous benefits, it also presents significant risks to our mental well-being.

Social media, in particular, has had an undeniable impact on mental health. What was once a platform for connecting with friends has transformed into a space that often dictates how we perceive ourselves and others. The need for validation through likes, shares, and comments can exacerbate feelings of insecurity and anxiety. The pressure to curate an idealized version of life for online consumption can leave people feeling inadequate, contributing to a growing sense of loneliness and depression.

Smartphones, another central element of digital dependency, have become both a blessing and a curse. On one hand, they provide instant access to information and keep us connected to the world at all times. On the other hand, they are a constant source of distraction and stress. The addiction to screen time is a growing concern, with individuals spending hours each day scrolling through feeds, watching videos, or playing games. This overexposure to screens has been linked to issues like sleep deprivation, decreased productivity, and heightened levels of anxiety, leading to a complex relationship between technology and mental health.

The Rise of Social Media and Its Influence

The rise of social media has profoundly reshaped the way we communicate, form relationships, and even view ourselves. What began as a way to stay in touch with friends and family has transformed into a global phenomenon, influencing nearly every aspect of modern life. Platforms like Facebook, Instagram, Twitter, TikTok, and others have revolutionized the way people interact with the world, offering opportunities for self-expression, connection, and business. However, beneath the surface of this digital revolution lies a host of psychological and social consequences that are often overlooked.

One of the most significant impacts of social media is its ability to amplify the desire for validation. With the rise of likes, comments, and shares, social media has introduced a new form of instant gratification. People are increasingly seeking approval from their online communities, whether through the number of likes on a photo or the comments on a post. This constant cycle of seeking external validation has led to a growing number of individuals experiencing feelings of inadequacy and low self-esteem, particularly among younger users. The more validation someone receives, the more they may feel compelled to share curated versions of their lives, often showcasing only the highlights. This can create a distorted view of reality, where people compare their everyday lives to the carefully filtered portrayals of others.

Social media has also contributed to a rise in mental health issues, particularly anxiety and depression. Research has shown that people who spend excessive amounts of time on social media are more likely to experience symptoms of these conditions. The pressure to maintain a certain image, the constant comparison to others, and the fear of missing out (FOMO) can all contribute to negative mental health outcomes. Social media's ability to keep users engaged by constantly bombarding them with new content has been linked to increased stress levels, as the brain struggles to keep up with the constant flow of information. This constant connectivity can also lead to social isolation, as people spend more time online and less time engaging in face-to-face interactions.

Another critical issue that has emerged with social media is the spread of misinformation. With millions of voices contributing to digital platforms, it has become increasingly difficult to distinguish between truth and falsehood. The rapid dissemination of false information can fuel fear, division, and confusion, further amplifying societal anxiety. In some cases, social media has been used as a tool to manipulate public opinion, as seen in the context of political campaigns and social movements.

Despite the undeniable advantages of social media—such as the ability to connect across geographical boundaries and the opportunity to create online communities—its impact on mental health cannot be ignored. The pressure to constantly engage, maintain a perfect image, and compare oneself to others has made social media a double-edged sword, where users must carefully navigate its influence on their well-being. As we continue to embrace the digital age, it is crucial to recognize and address the psychological effects of social media use and find ways to foster a healthier, more balanced relationship with these platforms.

Smartphones: A Double-Edged Sword for Mental Health

Smartphones have undeniably become an integral part of modern life, revolutionizing the way we communicate, access information, and manage daily tasks. With instant access to the internet, social media, and a host of other apps, smartphones provide unparalleled convenience and connectivity. However, their widespread use has led to significant consequences for mental health, positioning smartphones as a double-edged sword in our digital lives.

On one hand, smartphones have provided numerous benefits that can improve mental well-being. They allow for constant communication with loved ones, help users stay organized, and offer access to tools that can enhance productivity and mental stimulation. Apps designed for mental health, such as meditation tools, mood trackers, and mindfulness exercises, have become readily available, providing individuals with resources to manage stress, anxiety, and depression. Smartphones also enable access to online communities that can offer support and advice, particularly for those facing mental health challenges. In many ways, smartphones have made mental health resources more accessible than ever before.

On the other hand, the constant presence of smartphones in our lives can contribute to mental health struggles. The addiction to smartphones has become a growing concern, with individuals spending hours each day glued to their screens. This overuse can lead to a range of issues, including sleep disturbances, anxiety, and a decrease in overall well-being. One of the most significant problems linked to smartphone use is the constant exposure to notifications, which create a sense of urgency and disrupt our ability to focus. This constant bombardment of information can increase stress and overwhelm the brain, which struggles to process the sheer volume of data.

Moreover, the addictive nature of smartphones often results in people spending more time engaging with digital content than interacting with those around them. Social isolation can stem from excessive smartphone use, as individuals become absorbed in their devices, neglecting face-to-face interactions. This shift in communication patterns can lead to feelings of loneliness and disconnection, particularly in an age where virtual interactions often replace in-person relationships.

Another concern is the role of smartphones in exacerbating the comparison culture, particularly through social media platforms. Constant exposure to curated content and idealized versions of others' lives can negatively impact self-esteem. People often compare their own lives to the highlight reels presented by others, leading to feelings of inadequacy and frustration. The pressure to maintain an idealized online persona can create mental strain, contributing to anxiety and depression.

Finally, the overuse of smartphones has been linked to a phenomenon known as "technostress," a condition where the constant connectivity and information overload lead to burnout. Constantly being reachable via emails, messages, and social media can blur the lines between work and personal life, leaving individuals feeling perpetually "on" and unable to unwind. This lack of boundaries has a profound impact on mental health, particularly as it becomes increasingly difficult to find moments of peace and relaxation.

In summary, while smartphones offer undeniable advantages, they also come with significant mental health risks. The key lies in finding a balance between using smartphones to enhance life and recognizing when they begin to negatively impact our mental well-being. Through mindful use and setting healthy boundaries, individuals can mitigate the adverse effects and reap the benefits of these powerful devices.

The Addiction to Screen Time and Its Consequences

The addiction to screen time has become one of the most prevalent challenges of the digital age, impacting individuals of all ages and walks of life. With the rise of smartphones, tablets, computers, and smart TVs, people are now spending more time in front of screens than ever before. While screen time offers various benefits, such as entertainment, education, and connectivity, its excessive use has far-reaching consequences for mental and physical health.

One of the primary consequences of excessive screen time is the disruption of sleep patterns. Studies have shown that prolonged exposure to screens, especially before bedtime, can negatively affect sleep quality. The blue light emitted from screens interferes with the body's natural production of melatonin, the hormone that regulates sleep. As a result, individuals may experience difficulty falling asleep, insomnia, or poor-quality sleep. Lack of sleep can lead to increased stress, decreased cognitive function, mood swings, and long-term health issues such as heart disease, obesity, and weakened immune systems.

Another significant impact of screen addiction is the increase in anxiety and stress. The constant influx of notifications, messages, and updates from social media and other platforms can create a sense of urgency and pressure to remain constantly connected. This "always-on" mindset can lead to heightened stress levels, as individuals feel the need to respond to messages, check emails, or scroll through feeds at all hours of the day. Furthermore, social media platforms exacerbate this issue by creating an environment of comparison, where individuals compare their own lives to the seemingly perfect, curated lives of others. This leads to feelings of inadequacy, loneliness, and dissatisfaction, all of which contribute to anxiety and depression.

Physical health is also affected by excessive screen time. Prolonged sitting in front of a screen contributes to sedentary lifestyles, which are linked to a range of health issues, including obesity, cardiovascular problems, and poor posture. The lack of physical activity and prolonged screen use can also lead to musculoskeletal issues, such as neck and back pain, commonly referred to as "tech neck." Additionally, eye strain is a common complaint, as staring at a screen for long periods without taking breaks can lead to discomfort, blurred vision, and headaches, collectively known as digital eye strain.

The addictive nature of screen time also interferes with personal relationships and social interactions. As individuals become absorbed in their screens, they may spend less time engaging in face-to-face interactions with friends and family. This can lead to feelings of isolation and loneliness, even as individuals are constantly connected online. The lack of meaningful, in-person communication can erode the quality of relationships, contributing to emotional disconnection and social anxiety.

Moreover, the addiction to screen time impacts productivity. While technology offers various tools to enhance productivity, excessive screen time can lead to procrastination, distractions, and a lack of focus. Individuals may find it difficult to concentrate on tasks, especially as they are constantly drawn to their phones or computers for entertainment or social interaction.

The addiction to screen time has serious consequences for both mental and physical health. While screens are an essential part of modern life, it is crucial to establish boundaries and engage in mindful screen usage to prevent these negative effects. Finding a balance between screen time and offline activities, such as physical exercise, socializing, and relaxation, is key to maintaining overall well-being in the digital age.

Chapter 2
The Mental Health Crisis: A Global Perspective

The mental health crisis has become a global concern, with increasing rates of anxiety, depression, and other mental health disorders, particularly among youth. The rise of digital technology and social media, combined with modern-day pressures, has created a perfect storm for the deterioration of mental well-being, especially in younger generations. Social media platforms, constant connectivity, and the relentless pressure to maintain an idealized online persona have amplified existing challenges for young people, making it harder to navigate the complexities of identity, self-worth, and emotional stability.

The growing prevalence of anxiety and depression among youth is alarming, and while many factors contribute to these issues, the impact of digital culture cannot be ignored. In an era where young people are exposed to a constant stream of curated images and content, the pressure to compare oneself to others is ever-present. This comparison often leads to negative self-perception and heightened anxiety, which can manifest in a variety of ways, from social withdrawal to physical symptoms such as sleep disturbances.

As more research emerges, it becomes clear that social media plays a significant role in the escalation of these mental health issues. While these platforms offer opportunities for connection and self-expression, they also create environments where cyberbullying, unrealistic beauty standards, and a constant need for validation thrive. The constant flow of information, coupled with the fear of missing out (FOMO), exacerbates feelings of isolation and insecurity, leading to more severe mental health consequences.

Global studies on the intersection of technology and mental health provide valuable insights into the growing epidemic of mental health challenges. These studies reveal concerning trends, highlighting the widespread impact of screen time, social media engagement, and digital exposure on mental well-being. Understanding the global scope of this issue is essential for identifying effective solutions and raising awareness about the importance of mental health in the digital age.

Increased Anxiety and Depression Among Youth

The rise in anxiety and depression among youth has become one of the most concerning issues in today's society. While mental health challenges have always been present, the increasing prevalence of anxiety and depression in young people is undeniably alarming. This surge can be attributed to multiple factors, including societal pressures, changes in lifestyle, and, more significantly, the growing influence of technology and social media.

In recent years, studies have shown that anxiety and depression rates among adolescents and young adults have risen dramatically. The pressures associated with academic performance, social expectations, and future uncertainties have long been contributing factors, but the advent of digital technology has exacerbated these issues. Smartphones, social media, and the constant connectivity provided by the internet have created an environment where young people are constantly exposed to an overwhelming amount of information, much of which can be anxiety-inducing.

A major contributor to the rise in anxiety and depression among youth is the constant exposure to social media platforms. Social media has made it easier for young people to compare themselves to others, often leading to feelings of inadequacy and insecurity. The culture of "highlight reels" on platforms like Instagram, where only the best moments are shared, creates unrealistic expectations and fosters negative self-perception. Studies have found that those who spend more time on social media are more likely to report feelings of depression, loneliness, and low self-esteem. This phenomenon, known as social comparison, causes young people to measure their worth against the often idealized images presented by their peers or influencers.

Additionally, the "fear of missing out" (FOMO) has become a pervasive issue for young people navigating social media. The constant stream of updates from friends, family, and celebrities about their seemingly perfect lives can amplify feelings of isolation and anxiety. Young people may feel that they are not living up to the standards set by those they see online, leading to depression, particularly if they feel left out or disconnected from the activities being showcased on social media.

Furthermore, the pressures of academic achievement and the fear of not meeting societal expectations contribute to increasing levels of stress and anxiety among youth. The high expectations placed on young people to excel academically, socially, and eventually professionally have created an environment where failure is often perceived as devastating. This fear of failure, combined with an overwhelming sense of being constantly judged, is a breeding ground for anxiety and depression.

The constant use of smartphones and digital devices has also contributed to a decrease in face-to-face interactions, which are vital for emotional development and social bonding. The more young people turn to screens for entertainment, social interaction, or validation, the less likely they are to engage in meaningful, offline relationships. This isolation can further fuel feelings of loneliness, deepening the cycle of depression and anxiety.

The increasing rates of anxiety and depression among youth are influenced by a complex combination of factors, with technology and social media playing a significant role. The impact of constant connectivity, social comparison, and unrealistic standards of success has created a challenging environment for young people to navigate. Addressing this mental health crisis requires not only supporting youth in managing these digital pressures but also fostering environments that encourage self-acceptance, healthy coping mechanisms, and genuine human connections.

Social Media's Role in Escalating Mental Health Issues

Social media has undoubtedly transformed how people communicate, share experiences, and connect with others. However, its impact on mental health, particularly among youth, has raised significant concerns. While social media platforms provide a space for self-expression, creativity, and networking, they also foster environments that can escalate mental health issues, such as anxiety, depression, and low self-esteem.

One of the primary ways social media contributes to mental health struggles is through the culture of comparison. Social media platforms, by design, encourage individuals to present curated versions of their lives, often highlighting the most exciting, successful, or glamorous moments. This creates an environment where users are constantly exposed to the seemingly perfect lives of others. For young people, this is particularly harmful, as they are in the process of developing their self-identity. Seeing others' successes, travels, relationships, or achievements can lead to feelings of inadequacy or jealousy, as they may feel their own lives do not measure up to the idealized images they encounter online. Over time, these feelings of comparison can lead to lower self-worth, which is a key contributor to anxiety and depression.

Additionally, social media's emphasis on likes, comments, and other forms of validation creates a cycle of dependence on external approval. The act of posting a photo or sharing a status can trigger the desire for immediate feedback, often in the form of likes or comments. When the response is not as positive or immediate as expected, individuals may experience disappointment or anxiety. The pursuit of social validation becomes a constant cycle, with individuals feeling pressure to maintain an idealized version of themselves online. This pressure to perform and be validated can contribute to chronic stress and anxiety.

The phenomenon of cyberbullying has also become an unfortunate side effect of the social media age. The anonymity provided by the internet allows for harmful behavior that may not otherwise occur in face-to-face interactions. Harassment, name-calling, and the spread of rumors are rampant on many social platforms. Victims of cyberbullying often experience profound emotional distress, with lasting effects on their mental health. The constant fear of being targeted online can lead to feelings of powerlessness, fear, and depression, significantly impacting self-esteem and emotional well-being.

Another issue that social media exacerbates is the "fear of missing out" (FOMO). As individuals scroll through endless updates from friends, celebrities, or influencers, they may feel left out of exciting events, social gatherings, or opportunities. The perception that everyone else is living a better or more fulfilling life can deepen feelings of isolation and loneliness. This sense of missing out can create a constant state of anxiety and dissatisfaction, further fueling mental health problems.

Moreover, the constant exposure to negative news, distressing content, and divisive debates on social media can contribute to heightened stress levels. The news cycle on social platforms is often relentless, with stories of tragedy, violence, or political unrest dominating feeds. While staying informed is important, the constant bombardment of negative content can lead to information overload, anxiety, and a feeling of helplessness.

In summary, while social media can foster connection and provide a platform for self-expression, it also plays a significant role in escalating mental health issues. The culture of comparison, the need for validation, the prevalence of cyberbullying, and the constant exposure to negative content all contribute to the growing mental health crisis. To address these issues, individuals must develop healthier relationships with social media, set boundaries for online engagement, and prioritize self-care to protect their mental well-being.

Global Studies: What the Data Reveals

Global studies on the intersection of mental health and social media have provided valuable insights into how technology impacts well-being, particularly among youth. With rising concerns over the mental health crisis, researchers have delved into the role digital platforms play in exacerbating anxiety, depression, and other mental health issues. The data from these studies reveals troubling trends, demonstrating the widespread influence of social media and screen time on mental health across various demographics.

One significant finding from global studies is the correlation between increased screen time and mental health challenges. Research conducted by the Royal Society for Public Health (RSPH) in the UK found that young people who spend more than two hours a day on social media are more likely to experience mental health issues, including anxiety and depression. This is particularly true for platforms like Instagram, which encourages social comparison. A 2017 study from the University of Pennsylvania showed that limiting social media use to just 30 minutes per day led to significant reductions in depression and loneliness, highlighting the detrimental effects of prolonged exposure to digital platforms.

Global studies also suggest that the impact of social media on mental health is not uniform. Factors such as age, gender, and socio-economic status influence how individuals are affected by digital engagement. For example, studies have shown that adolescent girls are particularly vulnerable to the negative effects of social media, as they are more likely to internalize societal beauty standards and engage in upward social comparison. The constant exposure to idealized body images on platforms like Instagram has been linked to lower self-esteem and higher rates of body dissatisfaction among young women. This, in turn, can lead to anxiety, depression, and even eating disorders.

Moreover, a growing body of research from the World Health Organization (WHO) indicates that the rise in mental health issues is not confined to Western countries alone. Studies in countries like India, China, and Brazil have found that social media use is linked to increased feelings of isolation, loneliness, and stress in young people. In non-Western cultures, the pressure to conform to societal norms, combined with the influence of globalized beauty standards, has made social media even more damaging. A 2020 study from the International Journal of Environmental Research and Public Health revealed that excessive social media use in adolescents across Asia led to a rise in mental health problems, with many participants reporting increased feelings of stress, anxiety, and depression.

One of the key findings from global research is the role of social media in exacerbating the "Fear of Missing Out" (FOMO), which is prevalent across many age groups. A study by the University of Michigan revealed that FOMO is strongly associated with social media use and that it is a significant predictor of loneliness and depressive symptoms. People constantly checking their feeds, seeing others attend social events or achieve life milestones, can feel left out, leading to feelings of inadequacy and emotional distress.

Finally, studies are also showing the potential benefits of social media, particularly when used to raise awareness about mental health. Campaigns and hashtags like #HereForYou and EndTheStigma have helped open up conversations around mental health, reducing stigma and encouraging young people to seek help. For some, online communities provide a sense of belonging and emotional support, especially for those who feel isolated in their offline lives. However, the balance between the positive and negative effects of social media remains delicate and depends largely on how it is used.

Global studies reveal a clear and concerning relationship between social media use and mental health issues. While social media can offer connections and resources, its negative impact—especially when overused or used in unhealthy ways—cannot be ignored. The data calls for a more nuanced understanding of the relationship between digital engagement and mental health, emphasizing the need for mindful usage, digital literacy, and greater support systems for young people navigating these platforms.

Chapter 3
The Illusion of Connection

In the age of digital connectivity, social media has promised to bring people closer together, enabling relationships to flourish across distances. However, this promise often masks a deeper, more complex reality. Despite the constant flow of communication and interaction, social media frequently fosters superficial connections rather than genuine relationships. The very platforms designed to connect us have, in many cases, led to more isolation, disconnection, and emotional strain, especially for younger generations.

Superficial interactions on social media are becoming the norm, where likes, comments, and shares replace meaningful conversations and in-depth connections. As we spend more time online, the depth of our relationships often diminishes, replaced by surface-level engagements that fail to fulfill our emotional needs. These interactions, though frequent, lack the authenticity and vulnerability that characterize true human connection, leaving individuals with a sense of emptiness despite the constant stream of digital communication.

The culture of "likes" and social validation on social media platforms exacerbates this issue. The more approval a post receives, the more value a person may place on their online presence. However, this dependence on external validation often comes at the cost of self-esteem. People begin to measure their worth based on how they are perceived by others, which can lead to feelings of inadequacy and anxiety when they do not receive the expected response.

Moreover, the ever-present fear of missing out (FOMO) has intensified with social media's pervasive nature. Seeing others' curated moments, social gatherings, or achievements can lead to feelings of isolation and anxiety. The constant comparison to seemingly perfect lives online can deepen the divide between our reality and the idealized images we encounter, creating an ongoing cycle of dissatisfaction.

In this chapter, we will explore how these superficial interactions, the pursuit of validation, and the anxiety of FOMO are shaping modern relationships and contributing to the mental health challenges we face today.

Superficial Interactions: How Social Media Alters Relationships

Social media, while designed to bring people closer together, has significantly altered the nature of relationships in both positive and negative ways. While it offers platforms for connecting with friends, family, and strangers across vast distances, the interactions it fosters are often shallow and fleeting, lacking the depth and authenticity that define strong, meaningful relationships. The ease of communication online has led to an over-reliance on digital interaction, causing many people to substitute face-to-face communication with superficial exchanges that fail to nourish emotional bonds.

One of the most noticeable effects of social media on relationships is the shift from personal, in-depth conversations to brief, transactional exchanges. Texting, commenting, liking, and sharing posts have become the dominant forms of communication, while face-to-face conversations, which encourage emotional connection and the development of empathy, are becoming less frequent. These quick interactions are convenient but lack the nuance and richness of in-person dialogue. When emotions or complex thoughts are reduced to a string of emojis or a short reply, the essence of genuine connection is lost. As a result, social media often contributes to a sense of emotional distance, even when individuals are constantly "connected."

The nature of relationships on social media also promotes a false sense of closeness. In many cases, people may have hundreds or even thousands of online "friends" or followers, but the reality is that many of these connections are merely superficial. Social media provides an illusion of connection without the depth of true interaction. Friendships and romantic relationships can appear stronger online due to carefully curated content that showcases the best parts of one's life. However, these digital representations of relationships often fail to reflect the complexities, vulnerabilities, and struggles that form the foundation of real-life connections. As a result, people can feel more isolated despite having a large number of online connections.

Moreover, social media's algorithm-driven content delivery, which prioritizes likes, shares, and comments, tends to foster one-dimensional relationships. In pursuit of validation, people may present only the most polished versions of themselves, omitting the authentic, imperfect aspects of their lives. This selective sharing distorts the reality of personal interactions and can lead to unhealthy comparisons, as individuals compare their own lives to the seemingly perfect personas of others. Over time, this can create a sense of dissatisfaction, as people begin to measure their own worth based on the quantity of likes or the number of followers they have, rather than the quality of their personal relationships.

The prevalence of superficial interactions on social media has led to a paradox: despite being constantly connected, many individuals feel more disconnected than ever. The absence of meaningful communication, emotional support, and genuine connection leaves many feeling lonely, misunderstood, or emotionally drained. As relationships become increasingly mediated through digital platforms, the ability to cultivate deep, trusting, and empathetic bonds in the real world becomes more challenging, highlighting the negative impact that superficial online interactions can have on mental and emotional well-being.

The Impact of "Likes" and Validation on Self-Esteem

The culture of "likes" and social validation on social media has profoundly reshaped how individuals perceive themselves and their self-worth. What began as a simple form of interaction, where users could express appreciation for posts, has now evolved into a critical measure of success, popularity, and value. The pursuit of likes, comments, and shares has become a central aspect of online engagement, influencing how people view themselves and how they interact with others. This quest for validation has far-reaching consequences on self-esteem, particularly among adolescents and young adults.

The most obvious impact of the "like" culture is its reinforcement of the idea that self-worth is tied to external approval. When a post receives many likes, it can boost the poster's sense of validation and self-confidence. Conversely, posts that do not garner as much attention may trigger feelings of inadequacy, rejection, or self-doubt. This constant feedback loop creates an environment where individuals are more focused on the number of likes or comments they receive than the intrinsic value of what they share. As a result, self-esteem becomes heavily dependent on external validation, rather than internal feelings of self-worth and authenticity.

This reliance on social validation is particularly detrimental to younger users, who are still in the process of developing their sense of identity. Adolescents and young adults are at a stage in their lives where peer approval plays a significant role in shaping their self-image. When they post content online, they often do so with the expectation of receiving likes and positive feedback. The pressure to conform to certain beauty standards or social norms in order to gain approval can lead to significant anxiety and a distorted sense of self. Over time, this pursuit of validation can erode their self-confidence, as they begin to base their worth on the responses of others, rather than their own values and achievements.

The psychological effects of seeking validation through likes also extend to mental health. The constant cycle of posting and seeking approval can lead to heightened anxiety, especially when expectations are not met. Research has shown that individuals who are heavily invested in social media validation often experience increased stress and symptoms of depression. The fear of being overlooked or ignored online can foster a sense of loneliness and social isolation. Furthermore, the pressure to maintain a certain online persona can lead to a disconnect between one's true self and the version presented on social media. This dissonance can cause confusion, emotional distress, and a lack of fulfillment, as individuals feel compelled to live up to a curated version of themselves that may not reflect their true identity.

The impact of likes on self-esteem also extends beyond individual posts to the broader experience of social comparison. Social media platforms encourage users to constantly measure their lives against those of others. The curated nature of online content, where people often showcase their best moments, accomplishments, and experiences, leads to unrealistic comparisons. This can cause individuals to feel that their lives are less interesting or successful in comparison, further contributing to diminished self-esteem. The fear of missing out (FOMO) exacerbates these feelings, as people see others participating in exciting events or achieving milestones, making them feel left out or inferior.

The culture of "likes" and external validation on social media has created a fragile sense of self-esteem, particularly among younger generations. By tying self-worth to online approval, individuals are more likely to experience anxiety, depression, and dissatisfaction with their lives. To mitigate these negative effects, it is essential to foster a healthier relationship with social media, focusing on self-acceptance and internal validation rather than external approval. This shift can help individuals build a stronger sense of self-worth, grounded in authenticity and self-compassion.

The Anxiety of Missing Out: FOMO and Its Effects

The phenomenon of "Fear of Missing Out" (FOMO) has become increasingly prevalent in the digital age, driven largely by the pervasive influence of social media. FOMO is characterized by the anxiety individuals experience when they perceive that others are engaging in enjoyable or rewarding experiences that they are not part of. This feeling of exclusion or inadequacy is intensified by the constant stream of curated content that social media platforms offer. As users scroll through endless posts of their peers attending events, traveling, or achieving milestones, they are faced with a sense of disconnection and longing. The anxiety stemming from FOMO is not just about missing out on social events but also extends to the fear of missing out on opportunities, personal growth, or status.

At its core, FOMO reflects a deep-seated fear of social exclusion. Social creatures by nature, humans seek belonging and connection. When we see others participating in activities or enjoying experiences we aren't involved in, it triggers feelings of insecurity and a perceived lack of value. Social media, by constantly showcasing the most exciting and glamorous aspects of others' lives, magnifies these feelings of exclusion. The images and stories shared on platforms like Instagram or Facebook rarely reflect the full reality of people's lives, instead presenting an idealized version that is often edited or curated to highlight success and happiness. This disparity between what we see online and our own lived experiences can make us feel left out or inadequate.

FOMO is particularly impactful on younger generations, as they are more likely to spend substantial amounts of time on social media platforms. Adolescents and young adults, still in the process of forming their identities and social connections, are highly sensitive to perceived social exclusion. When their peers appear to be leading more exciting or fulfilling lives, the anxiety of missing out can lead to feelings of depression, low self-esteem, and loneliness. In some cases, FOMO can even lead to compulsive behaviors, such as excessive checking of social media accounts or trying to participate in every social event, regardless of whether it's healthy or enjoyable for them.

Moreover, FOMO can impact productivity and overall well-being. The constant bombardment of "perfect" experiences on social media can create a sense of urgency and pressure to keep up. As individuals strive to be part of every event or trend, they may find it difficult to focus on their personal goals or current activities. This perpetual cycle of chasing external validation and experiences leads to mental exhaustion and burnout, as individuals fail to prioritize their well-being and authentic interests. Instead of enjoying the present moment, they become preoccupied with what they might be missing.

In addition to social and emotional effects, FOMO can also impact physical health. The anxiety and stress caused by constantly feeling like others are having more fulfilling lives can contribute to sleep disturbances, as individuals stay up late scrolling through their feeds, trying to keep up with what everyone else is doing. The inability to disconnect from social media platforms leads to overexposure, exacerbating feelings of inadequacy and stress.

FOMO is a powerful and pervasive force in today's digital landscape, fueled by the curated, often idealized portrayals of life shared on social media. Its effects can be deeply harmful to an individual's mental health, leading to anxiety, depression, and a distorted sense of self-worth. To combat FOMO, it is essential to develop a more balanced relationship with social media, focusing on self-acceptance and mindfulness. By reducing the comparison to others and cultivating a stronger sense of personal fulfillment, individuals can protect their mental health and find greater contentment in their own lives.

Chapter 4
Cyberbullying and Online Harassment

In the digital age, the internet has brought people closer together, creating opportunities for connection and communication across vast distances. However, it has also given rise to a darker side of human interaction: cyberbullying and online harassment. Unlike traditional bullying, which takes place in physical spaces, cyberbullying occurs through digital platforms, such as social media, online games, and messaging apps. It can take many forms, including threatening messages, social exclusion, spreading rumors, and posting hurtful comments or images. The anonymity provided by the internet often emboldens perpetrators, making it easier for them to target their victims without facing the immediate consequences of face-to-face confrontation.

The prevalence of cyberbullying has surged in recent years, particularly among adolescents and young adults. Social media platforms, where people share their lives and personal stories, have become breeding grounds for harmful behavior. While many individuals use these platforms for positive connections, the constant connectivity has also made it easier for bullies to infiltrate victims' lives, often causing long-lasting psychological and emotional harm. Victims of cyberbullying can experience feelings of isolation, fear, and vulnerability, which can significantly impact their mental health.

The psychological consequences of online abuse are severe and can be just as damaging as those of traditional bullying. The anonymity of the internet can lead to more aggressive behavior, and the lack of face-to-face interaction can make it more difficult for victims to seek help or defend themselves. Cyberbullying can contribute to feelings of anxiety, depression, low self-esteem, and in some cases, suicidal ideation. The emotional toll of being relentlessly targeted online can have far-reaching effects on a person's mental and emotional well-being.

This chapter will explore the prevalence of cyberbullying in today's digital world, the psychological consequences of online abuse, and strategies for combating this growing issue. Understanding the impact of cyberbullying is crucial in order to develop effective solutions and protect vulnerable individuals in the digital space.

The Prevalence of Cyberbullying in the Digital World

The prevalence of cyberbullying has become a critical concern in the digital world, affecting individuals across various age groups, particularly adolescents and young adults. As digital technology and social media continue to permeate everyday life, the risk of online harassment has increased significantly. What makes cyberbullying particularly dangerous is its anonymity and reach—perpetrators can often hide behind fake profiles or remain unidentified, allowing them to target their victims without fear of immediate repercussion. Additionally, the 24/7 nature of the internet means that cyberbullying can occur at any time, intensifying the emotional and psychological distress experienced by victims.

Research has shown that cyberbullying is widespread, with millions of young people being affected globally. According to a 2019 study by the Cyberbullying Research Center, about one in five students in the United States reported being bullied online. This statistic has remained consistent across various studies and regions, indicating that cyberbullying is not a localized problem but a widespread issue with far-reaching consequences. The problem is not confined to one country or community but affects people from all walks of life. Social media platforms like Facebook, Instagram, Twitter, and newer platforms like TikTok have become hotspots for online harassment, where cyberbullies can target others through direct messages, comments, or public posts.

One of the reasons cyberbullying has become so prevalent is the growing dependence on social media for social interaction. Young people, in particular, use these platforms not only to connect with friends and family but also to define their identities, share experiences, and seek validation. However, the same platforms that offer these opportunities for self-expression have also exposed users to new forms of bullying. The speed at which harmful content can spread on social media contributes to the rapid escalation of online harassment. What might begin as a single hurtful comment or a meme shared with a few people can quickly snowball, reaching a much larger audience and inflicting lasting emotional damage on the victim.

The anonymity of the digital world makes cyberbullying even more prevalent. The lack of face-to-face interaction allows perpetrators to engage in harmful behaviors without the fear of immediate consequences. In many cases, they believe that they will not be caught or held accountable for their actions. This anonymity emboldens bullies, making it easier for them to target victims with impunity. The fact that cyberbullying can take place in private spaces—through direct messages or private groups—adds to its damaging nature. Victims often feel trapped and isolated, unable to escape the harassment even in the privacy of their own homes.

The prevalence of cyberbullying also varies depending on the platform and the individual's online activity. Studies have shown that young people who are more active on social media, particularly those who frequently share personal details or photos, are more likely to become victims of cyberbullying. Similarly, individuals who engage in online gaming or chat rooms may be at greater risk, as these spaces can foster hostile environments where harassment can flourish.

The prevalence of cyberbullying in the digital world has reached alarming levels, affecting millions of individuals, particularly youth. The combination of social media's widespread use, the anonymity provided by the internet, and the 24/7 nature of digital communication makes cyberbullying a pervasive issue. Addressing this problem requires a concerted effort from society, educators, and online platforms to raise awareness, promote responsible digital behavior, and implement policies to protect vulnerable individuals from online abuse.

Psychological Consequences of Online Abuse

The psychological consequences of online abuse, including cyberbullying, can be profound and long-lasting. Unlike traditional bullying, where the victim can escape by physically distancing themselves from the abuser, the nature of online abuse makes it difficult to avoid. The constant accessibility of social media and digital platforms means that the abuse can continue 24/7, causing emotional and mental distress that extends far beyond the virtual world and often manifests in real-life consequences.

One of the most immediate psychological effects of online abuse is increased anxiety. Victims of cyberbullying often experience heightened levels of stress and worry, constantly fearing the next instance of harassment. The fear of being targeted or ridiculed online can lead to hypervigilance, where individuals feel the need to constantly monitor their social media accounts, looking for signs of new attacks or negative comments. This anxiety can spiral, making it difficult to focus on daily tasks or enjoy activities, and in severe cases, it may lead to panic attacks or other anxiety disorders.

Depression is another common psychological consequence of online abuse. Victims often internalize the hurtful comments, exclusion, or rumors spread about them, leading to a sense of hopelessness and sadness. The emotional toll of being constantly belittled or humiliated online can cause feelings of worthlessness. Many victims of cyberbullying experience a decline in self-esteem as they become fixated on the negative feedback they receive. The inability to escape the online harassment leads to a pervasive sense of despair, and in some cases, it can contribute to suicidal thoughts or attempts.

The social isolation resulting from online abuse further compounds the emotional distress. Many victims of cyberbullying withdraw from social interactions, either to avoid further online harassment or because they feel stigmatized or ashamed. The fear of being judged or ridiculed can make it difficult for victims to engage in face-to-face interactions, which exacerbates feelings of loneliness. For young people, the fear of exclusion from social groups or online communities can lead to an increased sense of isolation, as social media platforms are often where they form and maintain relationships.

In addition to anxiety and depression, victims of online abuse often suffer from a loss of trust in others. Cyberbullying can shatter a person's sense of security and safety, both online and offline. As the abuse continues, victims may begin to view the online world as hostile, where others are untrustworthy or even malicious. This distrust can carry over into real-life relationships, leading to difficulties in forming healthy, supportive connections.

The psychological effects of online abuse can also manifest physically. The stress and emotional turmoil caused by being bullied online can lead to sleep disturbances, including insomnia, nightmares, and difficulty relaxing. Chronic stress can weaken the immune system, making victims more susceptible to illness. Additionally, some victims may experience physical symptoms like headaches, stomach aches, or unexplained fatigue, which are common psychosomatic responses to emotional stress.

Furthermore, the effects of online abuse are not always immediately apparent. In many cases, victims may hide the emotional scars from friends, family, or peers, out of fear of being judged or not being taken seriously. The shame and embarrassment associated with being targeted online often prevent individuals from seeking help or confiding in others. As a result, the psychological impact of online abuse can linger, sometimes for years, affecting a person's mental health, self-esteem, and overall quality of life.

In conclusion, the psychological consequences of online abuse are severe and multifaceted. Anxiety, depression, social isolation, and a loss of trust are just a few of the emotional tolls that victims face. The enduring nature of online harassment makes it particularly harmful, as it continuously disrupts a victim's mental health and well-being. Addressing these consequences requires greater awareness, supportive interventions, and stronger policies to protect individuals from online abuse and help victims heal.

Strategies for Combating Cyberbullying

Combating cyberbullying requires a multi-faceted approach involving individuals, families, schools, communities, and policymakers. The digital environment, with its anonymity and widespread access, makes cyberbullying a complex issue that demands comprehensive strategies for prevention, intervention, and support for victims. Effective strategies not only aim to reduce the incidence of online abuse but also focus on creating a safer, more supportive online environment.

One of the first and most important strategies for combating cyberbullying is **education and awareness**. Educating both children and adults about the nature of cyberbullying, its potential impact, and how to respond is crucial. Schools, parents, and communities need to foster discussions about responsible online behavior, the consequences of online harassment, and the importance of empathy and kindness in digital interactions. Social media platforms and online services can also play a role by providing resources and campaigns to educate users about cyberbullying and encouraging respectful online communication.

Open communication is another key strategy. Victims of cyberbullying often suffer in silence, either out of shame, fear, or lack of awareness of how to seek help. Therefore, creating an environment where young people feel comfortable talking about their experiences is essential. Parents, educators, and mentors should encourage open, non-judgmental conversations about the challenges young people face online. When individuals feel safe and supported, they are more likely to report instances of cyberbullying, enabling timely intervention.

Another crucial strategy is **monitoring and setting boundaries** around internet use. Parents and guardians can play a significant role by monitoring their children's online activities. While this does not mean invading their privacy, it involves having conversations about which platforms they use, who they interact with, and the kind of content they engage with. Setting time limits on screen use can also help reduce exposure to harmful content, while creating a healthy balance between online and offline activities. Schools and educational institutions can also set up monitoring systems to detect instances of online bullying among students, especially on school-related platforms.

Encouraging digital literacy and resilience is also a vital part of combating cyberbullying. Digital literacy equips individuals with the skills to navigate online spaces safely and responsibly. It also empowers them to recognize online abuse and understand how to protect themselves from it. Teaching young people how to block, report, and handle abusive messages or comments is key to giving them the tools they need to protect themselves. Additionally, promoting resilience through emotional intelligence programs and teaching coping strategies can help young people handle the emotional impact of online bullying. By fostering a sense of self-worth and emotional strength, individuals are better able to confront cyberbullying without being severely affected by it.

In terms of intervention, it is critical that those who experience or witness cyberbullying know how to report it. Many social media platforms and websites have built-in tools to report abuse, which should be utilized as a first step in dealing with harassment. In cases of severe bullying, intervention from professionals, such as school counselors, mental health experts, or legal authorities, may be necessary. Law enforcement can intervene when cyberbullying involves threats of violence, stalking, or other illegal activities, and legal measures can be taken to hold perpetrators accountable.

Finally, support for victims is an integral part of combating cyberbullying. Victims of cyberbullying often experience profound emotional distress, including anxiety, depression, and social isolation. Offering support through counseling, peer support groups, and mental health resources can help victims heal and regain their confidence. Schools and workplaces should have clear anti-bullying policies and support systems in place to provide assistance for victims of cyberbullying.

Combating cyberbullying requires a comprehensive, collaborative approach that involves education, communication, monitoring, intervention, and support. By creating a culture of respect, providing tools for self-protection, and offering a strong support network for victims, we can help reduce the prevalence of cyberbullying and mitigate its negative impact on mental health.

Chapter 5
The Role of Digital Detox in Mental Health

In today's hyper-connected world, technology has become an inseparable part of daily life. From social media notifications to work emails, screens are constantly demanding our attention, often leaving little room for respite. As a result, many individuals are experiencing burnout, stress, and mental fatigue due to the constant barrage of information. This has given rise to the concept of a **digital detox**—a conscious effort to unplug from digital devices and disconnect from the online world for a period of time.

Unplugging from screens is not just a temporary escape but an essential practice for mental wellness. The constant exposure to digital content can overstimulate the brain, contributing to increased levels of anxiety, stress, and feelings of being overwhelmed. A digital detox offers a much-needed break from this overstimulation, allowing individuals to recharge and refocus on real-life interactions and activities. In a world where people are increasingly defined by their online presence, taking time to step back can provide clarity, reduce stress, and help individuals reclaim their mental well-being.

Starting a digital detox may seem daunting, especially for those who are accustomed to being constantly connected. However, with practical steps and the right mindset, it is entirely achievable. Whether it's limiting social media use, setting aside designated "phone-free" times, or even taking a weekend off from all devices, the key is to create intentional boundaries that allow for more presence and mindfulness in daily life.

The long-term benefits of reduced screen time are profound. Not only does it help to reduce anxiety and improve focus, but it also nurtures healthier relationships, better sleep patterns, and overall emotional stability. This chapter will explore the importance of digital detox, provide actionable tips for getting started, and highlight the long-term mental health benefits of unplugging from the digital world.

Why Unplugging is Essential for Mental Wellness

In an increasingly digital world, the need to unplug and take breaks from screens has never been more crucial for mental wellness. While technology offers numerous benefits, such as staying connected, accessing information, and enhancing productivity, constant exposure to digital devices can take a toll on our mental and emotional well-being. This is why unplugging is essential for maintaining a healthy balance and safeguarding our mental health.

The constant bombardment of information from smartphones, social media, emails, and notifications can overwhelm the brain. Our minds are not equipped to process such an enormous amount of stimuli continuously. This overstimulation leads to heightened stress and anxiety, as the brain struggles to keep up with the relentless pace of information. It can also lead to what is commonly referred to as "information overload," where an individual feels mentally exhausted and unable to focus on any one task. This feeling of being constantly "on" leads to burnout, which can have a lasting impact on one's mental health and productivity.

Social media, in particular, contributes significantly to the need for unplugging. Platforms like Instagram, Facebook, and Twitter often present idealized versions of life, which can foster unhealthy comparisons and feelings of inadequacy. Constantly checking for likes, comments, or new posts can reinforce a sense of dependence on external validation, causing an erosion of self-esteem. Moreover, the fear of missing out (FOMO) can heighten feelings of anxiety and loneliness, as individuals see others seemingly leading more exciting or fulfilling lives. The emotional toll of this continuous connection to the virtual world can undermine mental wellness, especially among young people.

Additionally, excessive screen time disrupts other important aspects of mental health, such as sleep. Research has shown that exposure to blue light from screens interferes with the production of melatonin, the hormone responsible for regulating sleep. The result is disrupted sleep patterns, which can lead to fatigue, irritability, and difficulty concentrating. Chronic sleep deprivation is closely linked to a range of mental health problems, including anxiety, depression, and cognitive decline.

Unplugging from digital devices allows individuals to reset mentally, reduce stress, and reconnect with the present moment. Taking time off from screens fosters mindfulness, allowing for improved focus and clarity. Moreover, unplugging gives individuals the space to engage in offline activities, such as physical exercise, creative hobbies, and face-to-face interactions, all of which are essential for mental well-being.

Unplugging is essential for mental wellness because it helps to alleviate the stress, anxiety, and fatigue caused by constant digital stimulation. Taking breaks from technology allows individuals to regain mental clarity, focus, and emotional balance. It fosters healthier relationships, improves sleep, and provides the opportunity for self-reflection and personal growth. By embracing moments of disconnection, individuals can prioritize their mental health and achieve a more balanced and fulfilling life.

How to Start a Digital Detox: Practical Tips

Starting a digital detox can feel overwhelming, especially in a world where digital devices are deeply ingrained in daily life. However, taking the first steps towards unplugging can lead to significant improvements in mental well-being, productivity, and overall happiness. A digital detox is essentially about creating intentional boundaries between yourself and the digital world. One of the simplest ways to begin a digital detox is by setting clear limits on your screen time. Start by identifying specific periods in the day when you want to avoid screens. For example, designate the first hour after waking up and the last hour before bed as "screen-free" times. During these hours, focus on activities like reading, exercising, meditating, or spending time with loved ones. Setting boundaries around screen time helps reduce the constant checking of notifications and emails, allowing you to create space for more meaningful activities.

Constant notifications are one of the leading causes of digital overstimulation. The persistent pings and alerts can make it difficult to focus, leading to stress and anxiety. A simple yet effective way to begin your digital detox is by turning off non-essential notifications. For example, disable notifications for social media apps, news outlets, and shopping apps that aren't urgent. This minimizes distractions and allows you to focus on the present moment without being interrupted by digital noise.

Another great way to unplug is by creating designated "technology-free zones" in your home or workspace. For instance, make the dining table, bedroom, and living room spaces where phones, tablets, and computers are not allowed. This helps to create boundaries between your online and offline worlds and promotes healthier habits, such as engaging in face-to-face interactions, enjoying meals without distractions, and getting better sleep without the temptation of checking screens before bed.

If you find it challenging to disconnect on a daily basis, consider committing to a full digital detox day each week. Choose a day, like a Saturday or Sunday, to stay offline completely. Use this time to reconnect with hobbies, explore nature, enjoy time with family and friends, or engage in creative activities like writing, painting, or cooking. A weekly detox day will help you create a routine that prioritizes physical and mental well-being, offering a regular break from the pressure of the digital world.

One of the challenges of starting a digital detox is filling the void left by screen time. To avoid feeling bored or disconnected, replace your digital habits with offline activities that nourish your mind and body. Engage in activities like exercising, practicing mindfulness or meditation, cooking, gardening, journaling, or reading. By making these activities a regular part of your day, you can shift your focus away from the digital world and enhance your sense of fulfillment and presence.

Social media can be a major source of digital stress and anxiety. While it's difficult to completely avoid, a digital detox doesn't mean you have to disconnect entirely from social media. Instead, try to be more mindful of how and when you use it. Limit your social media time to a set amount each day, and unfollow accounts that contribute to negative emotions or self-comparisons. Prioritize accounts that bring positivity, inspiration, or helpful information, and avoid mindlessly scrolling through your feeds.

Ironically, technology can help facilitate your digital detox. There are numerous apps available that can help you track your screen time, limit your app usage, or even block distracting websites. Apps like "Forest," "Moment," or "Screen Time" can help you stay on track by reminding you when you've reached your set screen limits or by encouraging you to stay offline.

Starting a digital detox doesn't require drastic measures but rather small, intentional changes that gradually shift the focus from digital dependency to healthier, more balanced habits. Whether it's setting boundaries, reducing notifications, or scheduling dedicated time offline, the goal is to reconnect with yourself, others, and the world around you. By practicing these tips, you can reclaim your time, reduce stress, and ultimately improve your mental and emotional health.

The Long-Term Benefits of Reduced Screen Time

Reducing screen time, particularly in the age of constant digital engagement, offers numerous long-term benefits for mental, physical, and emotional well-being. While many people feel that their digital lives are a necessary part of modern existence, it's essential to recognize that minimizing screen time can have significant positive effects on overall health, relationships, and personal development.

One of the most notable long-term benefits of reduced screen time is improved mental health. Constant exposure to screens, particularly social media, is linked to an increase in anxiety, depression, and stress. By cutting down on screen time, individuals are less likely to engage in social comparison, which is often exacerbated by idealized portrayals of other people's lives on platforms like Instagram or Facebook. Without the constant barrage of notifications and pressure to present a curated version of life online, people often experience a reduction in feelings of inadequacy and loneliness. Over time, this leads to a healthier mindset, where self-worth is no longer defined by online validation but by real-life experiences and personal achievements.

Better sleep quality is another significant benefit of reducing screen time. Research has shown that the blue light emitted from screens interferes with the body's production of melatonin, the hormone responsible for regulating sleep cycles. Extended screen use, particularly before bed, disrupts sleep patterns, leading to insomnia, poor sleep quality, and daytime fatigue. By cutting down on screen time, especially in the evening, individuals can significantly improve their sleep. The long-term result is better physical and mental recovery during sleep, which is essential for cognitive function, emotional regulation, and overall health.

Moreover, reducing screen time can enhance productivity and focus. When people are less distracted by constant notifications, emails, and messages, they can concentrate better on tasks and engage in deeper work. Over time, this leads to more meaningful accomplishments, better time management, and greater satisfaction with personal and professional achievements. As people become less reliant on digital devices for entertainment and information, they often discover new hobbies and interests that don't involve screens, leading to a more fulfilling and well-rounded life.

Another benefit of reducing screen time is improved physical health. Excessive screen time often leads to a sedentary lifestyle, with many people spending hours sitting in front of computers, smartphones, or televisions. This can contribute to issues such as obesity, poor posture, eye strain, and even cardiovascular problems. Reducing screen time encourages more physical activity, whether it's walking, exercising, or simply engaging in non-screen-based activities. Over time, this leads to better cardiovascular health, improved posture, and a reduced risk of chronic diseases such as diabetes and heart disease.

Finally, reducing screen time strengthens real-world connections. In a digital world, face-to-face interactions are increasingly rare, and relationships can suffer as a result. By cutting back on screen time, individuals have more opportunities to connect with family, friends, and peers in person. Meaningful, in-person interactions foster stronger bonds, improve communication skills, and enhance emotional intimacy. The long-term result is healthier relationships, greater social support, and a deeper sense of belonging.

Chapter 6
The Effects of Constant Information Overload

In today's world, we are constantly surrounded by an influx of information. From 24/7 news cycles to social media updates, emails, and endless digital notifications, we are always connected and always informed—often to the point of overload. While technology has made access to information easier than ever before, it has also created an environment where it can feel impossible to escape the constant barrage of news, opinions, and updates. This overwhelming flow of information has profound psychological effects, leading to increased stress, anxiety, and a sense of being mentally fatigued.

The 24/7 news cycle is a major contributor to this information overload. With the rise of digital platforms, news is no longer confined to specific hours or scheduled broadcasts; it's now a continuous stream, constantly updating and often sensationalized. The relentless nature of the news cycle, especially with breaking news and crisis reporting, keeps people in a constant state of alertness. This, in turn, leads to heightened anxiety and stress, as individuals feel the need to stay informed at all times, even when the information is distressing or unnecessary. The constant intake of negative news can leave people feeling overwhelmed, helpless, and emotionally drained.

Moreover, navigating the stress of digital information consumption becomes more challenging as people struggle to filter what is essential from what is not. The sheer volume of digital content available makes it difficult to discern what is relevant or important, further contributing to cognitive overload.

In this chapter, we will explore the effects of constant information overload, focusing on how the 24/7 news cycle contributes to psychological strain, the challenges of managing digital consumption, and practical steps to find balance by curating your digital environment. Learning to manage the information we consume is critical for protecting our mental well-being in an era of constant connectivity.

The 24/7 News Cycle and Its Psychological Toll

The 24/7 news cycle has fundamentally changed how we consume information, making it a constant presence in our lives. Unlike the traditional news model of scheduled broadcasts, the rise of digital media and social platforms means that news is available at all times, in real-time, and often in an endless stream. While the constant flow of information can be useful for staying updated on current events, it also has significant psychological consequences. The relentless nature of the 24/7 news cycle has created an environment where individuals feel pressured to stay informed constantly, leading to increased stress, anxiety, and emotional fatigue.

One of the most profound psychological tolls of the 24/7 news cycle is the phenomenon of information overload. With the rapid and constant updates from various news outlets, it becomes difficult to process and filter what is truly important. The sheer volume of information—ranging from breaking news, global crises, and political unrest to celebrity gossip and social issues—can overwhelm the mind. People often feel compelled to keep up with every new headline, which leads to mental exhaustion. This information saturation makes it challenging for individuals to focus on anything for an extended period, as their minds are constantly shifting between different pieces of news and stories.

The negativity bias in the media also amplifies the psychological toll of the news cycle. News outlets are often more likely to report on negative or sensational stories, as these tend to capture more attention and drive higher engagement. This results in an overwhelming amount of distressing information being fed to the public. Whether it's reports of violence, political conflict, economic instability, or natural disasters, the consistent exposure to negative news can lead to fear, helplessness, and anxiety. Constantly hearing about global crises or personal tragedies can create a sense of uncertainty about the future and an ongoing feeling of doom. Over time, this constant barrage of negative information can contribute to anxiety disorders, depression, and even a sense of helplessness.

Another psychological effect of the 24/7 news cycle is news fatigue. The pressure to stay constantly informed can lead to burnout, where individuals begin to disengage from consuming news altogether. While some may initially feel anxious about not knowing what's happening in the world, others experience fatigue from the emotional toll of continuous exposure to distressing events. This mental exhaustion from staying constantly connected to the news cycle can lead to a feeling of being disconnected, overwhelmed, and emotionally drained, which affects productivity, relationships, and overall well-being.

Moreover, the 24/7 news cycle can disrupt sleep patterns, particularly for those who feel the need to check the news before going to bed. The exposure to high-stress stories or unsettling news right before sleep can increase anxiety levels and disrupt the ability to relax, leading to poor sleep quality. Sleep deprivation, in turn, has a compounding effect on mental health, as it exacerbates stress, mood swings, and cognitive impairments.

In summary, the 24/7 news cycle, while providing constant access to information, has serious psychological consequences. The continuous exposure to a deluge of news, often dominated by negativity and sensationalism, leads to increased stress, anxiety, and mental fatigue. To mitigate these effects, it is crucial to set boundaries around news consumption, limit exposure to distressing content, and engage in regular digital detoxes to protect mental well-being. Balancing information intake with periods of disconnection can help preserve emotional health and prevent burnout in an increasingly connected world.

Navigating the Stress of Digital Information Consumption

Navigating the stress of digital information consumption is becoming an increasingly important challenge in today's fast-paced, always-on world. With the constant flow of news, updates, notifications, and advertisements across multiple platforms, it can be difficult to manage the overwhelming amount of information we encounter daily. This constant bombardment can lead to information fatigue, where the sheer volume of digital content begins to take a toll on our mental health, making it harder to process and engage with information in a meaningful way.

One of the primary sources of stress in digital information consumption is the overload of stimuli. Whether it's news articles, social media updates, or work emails, the brain is forced to handle an enormous amount of content at once. Studies have shown that constantly switching between different types of information—work-related tasks, personal messages, and social media updates—can lead to cognitive overload. This overload diminishes our ability to focus and retain information, leaving us feeling mentally drained and unable to fully process what we're reading or watching. Over time, this can result in burnout and a sense of being constantly on edge.

Another major stressor of digital information consumption is the pressure to stay informed. In an era where breaking news is constantly available, there is an unspoken expectation to be aware of everything happening in the world. This pressure to remain updated, often fueled by social media, can contribute to anxiety and a feeling of being overwhelmed. People may feel guilty for not staying up to date on current events or for missing out on important trends or conversations. However, this constant need to consume information can be mentally exhausting, leaving little room for relaxation or personal reflection.

Additionally, the constant flow of negative or sensationalized content can significantly increase stress levels. News outlets often prioritize stories that generate strong emotional reactions, particularly those that are negative or alarming. The negativity bias inherent in digital media makes it easy to be flooded with distressing stories, such as political crises, natural disasters, or personal tragedies. Continuous exposure to such content can create a sense of helplessness, fear, and stress, as people internalize the challenges faced by others without feeling equipped to make a meaningful impact. This can contribute to a cycle of emotional depletion and anxiety.

To manage the stress of digital information consumption, intentional digital habits are essential. One effective strategy is to set time limits for how long you spend on information-consuming platforms each day. By reducing the time spent on news websites or social media, individuals can prevent themselves from being overwhelmed by constant updates. Another helpful tactic is to curate your digital environment by following only trusted, positive, or educational sources. Limiting exposure to sources that amplify negativity or sensationalism can help reduce stress. Additionally, creating designated "screen-free" times during the day—such as before bed or during meals—can help prevent information overload from disrupting your mental clarity and relaxation.

Finally, it's crucial to prioritize self-care and mental breaks. Taking time for activities that help decompress, such as meditation, physical exercise, or simply enjoying a hobby, can provide a much-needed escape from the digital world. These breaks help reset the brain and give individuals the space to recharge emotionally and mentally. Engaging in mindfulness practices can also help individuals become more aware of their reactions to digital content, allowing them to manage stress more effectively.

Finding Balance: Curating Your Digital Environment

Finding balance in today's digital world requires intentional effort and careful curation of the content and platforms we engage with. The sheer volume of information available at our fingertips can be overwhelming, and without actively managing what we consume, we risk experiencing mental burnout, anxiety, and stress. Curating your digital environment is about taking control over what enters your personal space online, ensuring that the content you encounter supports your well-being, productivity, and overall mental health.

The first step in curating your digital environment is understanding the impact of what you consume. Much of the content we encounter daily—whether through social media, news outlets, or online discussions—can shape our thoughts, emotions, and perspectives. Therefore, it's essential to evaluate the content we're exposed to and identify sources that may contribute to stress, negativity, or feelings of inadequacy. For instance, if scrolling through certain social media accounts or watching sensationalized news triggers anxiety or low self-esteem, it's important to limit exposure to those platforms. Instead, prioritize content that brings value, such as educational resources, positive news, or uplifting personal stories. Recognizing the influence of what you see and hear online is key to shaping a more positive digital experience.

Another strategy for curating your digital environment is organizing and controlling your social media feeds. Social media is often a major contributor to mental stress, especially with its tendency to showcase curated and idealized versions of others' lives. Begin by unfollowing or muting accounts that make you feel inadequate, jealous, or overwhelmed. Follow accounts that promote positivity, mental wellness, inspiration, or content related to your personal passions and interests. Social media platforms like Instagram, Facebook, and Twitter all allow users to tailor their experience by adjusting who they follow and what they see. By consciously curating your feed, you create an environment that nurtures self-growth and reduces exposure to negativity.

Additionally, turning off unnecessary notifications can significantly reduce the stress of constant digital engagement. Whether it's from email, social media, or news apps, notifications can interrupt your focus and keep your mind in a perpetual state of alertness. By turning off non-essential notifications, you regain control of when and how you engage with digital content. Instead of being at the mercy of pings and alerts, you can choose designated times to check messages, emails, and updates. This simple adjustment helps you reclaim your time and energy, fostering a more mindful approach to your digital interactions.

Another important aspect of curating your digital environment is setting boundaries around screen time. Establishing "tech-free" zones in your home or specific times during the day to disconnect from devices can help restore balance. For example, setting aside time before bed as a screen-free period not only improves sleep quality but also promotes relaxation and mindfulness. Creating these boundaries encourages healthier habits, such as spending more time outdoors, engaging in hobbies, or connecting with loved ones in person—activities that are essential for maintaining mental well-being.

Finally, curating your digital environment involves investing in tools that promote focus and productivity. Many apps and platforms are designed to help individuals manage their screen time, block distractions, and reduce digital clutter. Apps like "Forest," "Focus@Will," or "Freedom" can help minimize distractions, allowing you to stay focused on tasks that matter most. These tools support your effort to create a more intentional and balanced relationship with technology.

Finding balance in the digital world requires a proactive approach to curating the content and experiences we engage with. By understanding the impact of digital content, organizing social media feeds, limiting notifications, setting time boundaries, and using productivity tools, you can create a digital environment that supports mental well-being, focus, and overall life satisfaction. Taking control of your digital environment not only reduces stress but also empowers you to make intentional choices about how technology fits into your life.

Chapter 7
Mindfulness in the Digital Age

In the fast-paced, always-connected world of the digital age, maintaining mental well-being can be a challenge. The constant influx of information, notifications, and digital interactions can easily lead to stress, overwhelm, and burnout. Amid this digital noise, mindfulness offers a powerful tool for regaining balance, focus, and inner calm. Digital mindfulness, a concept that integrates traditional mindfulness practices with our modern digital lives, has emerged as a crucial strategy for managing the psychological toll of constant connectivity.

Digital mindfulness involves intentionally focusing on the present moment and cultivating awareness of one's thoughts, feelings, and reactions while engaging with technology. Unlike mindlessly scrolling through social media or hastily checking emails, digital mindfulness encourages conscious and deliberate interactions with digital content. By being more present in our digital interactions, we can reduce stress, avoid distractions, and foster healthier habits when using technology.

In this chapter, we will explore how mindfulness can help mitigate the stress caused by digital overload and how it can lead to a more intentional, fulfilling relationship with technology. We will discuss the benefits of practicing mindfulness in a world dominated by screens, including its ability to improve focus, reduce anxiety, and promote emotional well-being. Additionally, we will examine practical tools and techniques for integrating mindfulness into daily digital interactions, allowing individuals to better manage their time online and make intentional choices that support their mental health. By incorporating mindfulness into our digital lives, we can transform our relationship with technology, making it a tool for growth and well-being rather than a source of stress and distraction.

What Is Digital Mindfulness?

Digital mindfulness is the practice of applying traditional mindfulness principles to our digital interactions. In a world where we are constantly engaged with screens—whether it's checking emails, scrolling through social media, or consuming news—digital mindfulness offers a way to slow down and be more intentional about how we interact with technology. At its core, digital mindfulness is about cultivating awareness of the present moment while using digital devices, recognizing our emotional reactions, and making conscious choices about our digital behaviors.

Traditional mindfulness, a practice rooted in Buddhism and increasingly popular in Western psychology, involves focusing one's attention on the present moment without judgment. It encourages individuals to observe their thoughts, feelings, and bodily sensations with openness and curiosity. In the context of the digital world, this means being aware of how technology impacts our mental and emotional states and noticing when we are simply reacting to notifications, distractions, or information overload.

Digital mindfulness involves being intentional about how we engage with our devices and the content we consume. Instead of mindlessly scrolling through social media, watching endless videos, or checking our phones out of habit, digital mindfulness encourages us to be aware of our behavior and the emotional consequences of our online interactions. For example, instead of automatically reaching for your phone when you wake up, digital mindfulness suggests pausing and taking a moment to assess your mood, intentions, and what you truly need to focus on at that moment. This helps prevent the automatic and often reactive nature of digital engagement.

One of the primary goals of digital mindfulness is to create a healthier relationship with technology. In an era where constant notifications and the pressure to be always available can lead to burnout and anxiety, digital mindfulness helps individuals regain control over their time and attention. By practicing digital mindfulness, people can become more aware of their digital consumption habits and adjust them to reduce stress, promote well-being, and reclaim time for more meaningful offline activities. This approach enables individuals to set boundaries with technology and make intentional decisions about when, how, and why they engage with it.

How Mindfulness Can Help Mitigate Digital Stress

In a world where digital technology is an integral part of our daily lives, the constant flow of information, notifications, and virtual interactions can create a significant amount of stress. Digital stress, often fueled by information overload, social media pressure, and the expectation of being constantly connected, can lead to feelings of anxiety, burnout, and emotional exhaustion. Mindfulness, however, offers an effective way to mitigate this digital stress by fostering awareness, focus, and emotional regulation during digital interactions.

Mindfulness is the practice of being present and fully engaged in the moment, without judgment or distraction. By applying this practice to our digital interactions, we can gain better control over how we respond to the constant barrage of digital stimuli. Mindfulness encourages individuals to notice their physical and emotional reactions to digital content, allowing them to pause before reacting impulsively. This pause is crucial for managing the stress that often arises from the fast-paced nature of digital media, where emotions can be triggered in an instant by alarming news, contentious social media posts, or constant demands for attention.

One of the primary ways mindfulness mitigates digital stress is by promoting self-awareness. When we practice mindfulness, we become more attuned to our thoughts, feelings, and physical sensations. In the context of digital technology, this heightened self-awareness allows us to recognize when our digital habits are contributing to stress. For example, we may notice that certain activities, such as scrolling through social media or binge-watching videos, leave us feeling drained, anxious, or frustrated. With this awareness, we can make conscious choices about how to adjust our behavior—whether it's reducing screen time, limiting exposure to certain types of content, or taking breaks from devices.

Mindfulness also helps regulate emotional reactions to digital content. The digital world is often filled with highly charged, sensationalized material, which can evoke strong emotions like anger, sadness, or fear. By practicing mindfulness, we can become less reactive to these emotional triggers. Instead of automatically responding with frustration or anxiety, mindfulness helps us observe our emotional reactions without judgment and decide how to respond in a calm and measured way. This ability to pause and reflect helps prevent emotional burnout and promotes a sense of emotional balance even in the face of stressful digital interactions.

Another way mindfulness can mitigate digital stress is by encouraging intentionality in our use of technology. In a world where notifications and endless content demand our attention, it's easy to fall into the trap of mindless scrolling or multitasking. Mindfulness encourages us to be intentional with how we engage with digital devices, helping us prioritize our time and energy. For example, setting aside specific times for checking emails or social media, rather than reacting impulsively to every notification, allows us to control when and how we engage with technology. By being intentional with our digital consumption, we reduce the feeling of being overwhelmed by constant distractions.

Finally, mindfulness offers a way to reconnect with the present moment. Digital technology often pulls us out of the present moment, leading to a sense of detachment from our surroundings and relationships. Practicing mindfulness helps us re-anchor ourselves in the present, fostering a deeper connection with the world around us and reducing feelings of isolation or disconnection. When we are more present, we are less likely to feel distracted or overwhelmed by the digital world, leading to greater clarity, focus, and peace of mind.

Mindfulness is a powerful tool for mitigating digital stress. By promoting self-awareness, emotional regulation, intentional technology use, and presence in the moment, mindfulness helps us navigate the digital world with greater ease and balance. With mindfulness practices, individuals can reduce the negative effects of constant digital engagement and foster a healthier, more sustainable relationship with technology.

Tools and Techniques for Practicing Mindfulness Online

Practicing mindfulness in the digital age can be challenging due to the constant influx of information, notifications, and distractions from online platforms. However, there are several tools and techniques available that can help individuals integrate mindfulness practices into their online lives, reducing stress, increasing focus, and promoting overall mental well-being. One effective way to practice mindfulness is by using mindfulness apps. A wide range of apps are specifically designed to help individuals practice mindfulness and meditation in the digital world. These apps provide guided meditations, breathing exercises, and mindfulness reminders, making it easy to incorporate mindfulness into a busy lifestyle. Popular apps like Headspace, Calm, and Insight Timer offer meditation practices, sleep aids, and mindfulness techniques that can be used anywhere, anytime. These apps are great for beginners and experienced practitioners alike, offering a structured way to incorporate mindfulness into daily routines.

Mindfulness isn't just about meditation—it's also about being fully present in whatever task you're doing, whether it's working, studying, or interacting online. Focus apps like Forest, Freedom, or

StayFocusd can help reduce distractions by blocking certain websites or limiting the time spent on apps that cause you to drift away from your work or mindfulness practice. These tools help users focus on one task at a time, encouraging the practice of mindful productivity. By limiting interruptions, these tools create a conducive environment for being more present and engaged with tasks.

Social media is one of the most significant contributors to digital stress and information overload. However, it's possible to practice mindfulness while using social platforms. One approach is to curate your digital environment by unfollowing accounts or muting notifications that contribute to negative feelings, stress, or unnecessary distractions. Mindful scrolling involves paying full attention to what you are reading or engaging with and making conscious decisions about the content you consume. It can be helpful to set intentions before logging into social media, such as limiting time spent on platforms, focusing only on positive or informative content, or engaging with posts that genuinely contribute to your well-being.

Taking intentional breaks from screens is a vital mindfulness technique in an age dominated by digital consumption. Many devices and apps have built-in features to help you monitor and limit screen time, such as Apple's Screen Time or Android's Digital Wellbeing. These tools track how much time you spend on different apps, helping you become more aware of your digital habits. Setting daily limits for non-essential apps or implementing "screen-free" zones during the day (e.g., during meals or before bedtime) can help create mental space and promote mindfulness.

Online platforms can also be used to access resources that promote mindfulness through relaxation and breathing exercises. Websites like YouTube and apps like Breethe or Prana Breath offer guided deep breathing exercises, progressive muscle relaxation, and other mindfulness techniques that can help alleviate stress and promote calmness. By incorporating short, regular breathing breaks into your digital routine, you can reset your mind and emotions, helping you manage digital stress more effectively.

Practicing mindfulness can also be integrated into how we schedule and plan our online activities. By setting clear intentions for how we want to engage with digital platforms—whether for work, learning, or socializing—we can create a more intentional, mindful approach to using technology. Time-blocking techniques can help structure your day to allocate specific time slots for tasks, minimizing distractions and fostering focus. Apps like Trello, Google Calendar, or Notion can assist in organizing tasks and setting reminders for mindfulness activities, ensuring that mindfulness is embedded into your digital day.

Mindfulness can be practiced when engaging with online content, such as podcasts, videos, or webinars. Rather than passively consuming content, try to practice mindful listening and watching. This involves paying full attention to the content, noticing your thoughts and feelings as you consume information, and being present without judgment or multitasking. This type of engagement enhances the overall experience, leading to better retention and a deeper connection with the material.

Chapter 8
The Impact of Social Comparison on Mental Health

In the age of social media, our sense of self-worth has become increasingly intertwined with how we are perceived online. Platforms like Instagram, Facebook, and TikTok have given rise to a "highlight reel" culture, where individuals curate and share the best moments of their lives. While these platforms offer opportunities for connection and self-expression, they also foster a culture of comparison, where we often measure our lives against the idealized versions of others. The constant exposure to filtered images, achievements, and experiences shared by friends, influencers, and celebrities can significantly affect how we view ourselves.

The impact of this social comparison is profound, especially when it comes to mental health. Many individuals experience feelings of inadequacy, anxiety, and depression as a result of comparing their behind-the-scenes to the polished, curated lives of others. This type of comparison can distort reality, creating an unrealistic standard that is difficult to achieve or maintain. As a result, individuals may struggle with low self-esteem and diminished self-worth, constantly feeling like they fall short of societal expectations.

In this chapter, we will explore the psychological effects of social comparison, specifically focusing on how the "highlight reel" culture of social media contributes to negative self-perception. We will examine how comparison affects our mental health and self-worth, leading to anxiety and dissatisfaction. Finally, we will discuss strategies for breaking the cycle of harmful comparisons, including techniques to foster a healthier relationship with ourselves and a more balanced approach to social media use. By understanding the impact of social comparison and learning how to manage it, we can build a stronger, more positive sense of self in the digital age.

The "Highlight Reel" Culture of Social Media

The "highlight reel" culture of social media refers to the practice of selectively sharing only the most polished, glamorous, and successful moments of one's life while concealing the more mundane or challenging aspects. This culture, which thrives on platforms like Instagram, Facebook, and TikTok, fosters the illusion that everyone's life is exciting, perfect, and constantly filled with achievements. While social media allows individuals to connect with others and share experiences, it also creates a distorted reality where only the best moments are showcased, leaving out the behind-the-scenes struggles and imperfections that are part of every life.

The rise of the "highlight reel" culture has its roots in the desire to be seen and validated by others. As people post images of vacations, milestones, personal successes, and curated selfies, they seek positive reinforcement through likes, comments, and shares.

This curated perfectionism is often amplified by the algorithms that govern social media platforms, which prioritize posts that receive high engagement. As a result, individuals are encouraged to post only their most visually appealing and captivating content, further contributing to the cycle of showing only the "highlights" and not the full picture of their lives.

While this selective sharing may seem harmless on the surface, it can have significant psychological consequences. The constant exposure to other people's highlight reels can distort reality and create a sense of inadequacy. Users may start comparing their behind-the-scenes lives—marked by mundane routines, struggles, or failures—with the seemingly perfect lives of those they follow. This can lead to feelings of jealousy, disappointment, and self-doubt, especially when individuals perceive their lives as lacking in comparison to others' curated, idealized versions.

This "highlight reel" culture can also perpetuate unrealistic beauty standards, social norms, and life expectations. Images and videos on social media are often heavily edited, filtered, and staged to fit a certain aesthetic, further reinforcing unattainable ideals. The pressure to measure up to these standards can lead to a decline in self-esteem, body image issues, and a distorted sense of self-worth. The cycle of comparing one's life to others' curated, highlight-filled experiences can lead to anxiety, depression, and a lack of fulfillment, as people begin to equate their happiness and success with how they measure up against the idealized versions presented online.

In summary, the "highlight reel" culture of social media has created a warped sense of reality where only the best moments are showcased, leading to harmful social comparisons. The result is often a diminished sense of self-worth, as individuals struggle to reconcile their own experiences with the seemingly perfect lives of others. Recognizing the implications of this culture is key to developing a healthier, more balanced relationship with social media, one that celebrates authenticity and acknowledges the complexity of real life.

How Comparison Affects Our Self-Worth

Comparison is a natural human tendency; we often evaluate ourselves in relation to others as a way to make sense of our place in the world. However, in the age of social media, this tendency has been amplified, leading to significant impacts on our self-worth. When we compare ourselves to others—whether in terms of achievements, appearance, relationships, or lifestyle—we are engaging in a process that can either boost our confidence or erode it. Unfortunately, in a world where social media showcases an often idealized and selective version of people's lives, comparison more frequently leads to negative consequences for self-esteem and mental health.

When we compare our lives to the curated, "highlight reel" versions presented on social media, we tend to focus on the aspects of others' lives that we perceive as superior to our own. This type of comparison typically focuses on the outwardly visible elements— wealth, beauty, success, and happiness—which are often edited or staged. This skewed perspective can make us feel inadequate, as we measure our worth based on external factors that are not always representative of reality. For example, seeing a friend's vacation photos or a colleague's career achievements might prompt feelings of jealousy or inadequacy, leading us to believe that we are somehow less successful or fulfilled.

One of the most damaging effects of comparison is the internalization of these perceptions, which can directly influence how we view ourselves. Negative social comparisons can create a cycle of self-criticism and low self-esteem. When we feel that we are falling short compared to others, we may begin to devalue our own abilities, achievements, or personal qualities. Instead of recognizing our unique strengths and progress, we focus on our perceived flaws, believing that we are not measuring up to the standards set by others.

This constant comparison can also result in feelings of envy and discontent, which further erode our sense of self-worth. For example, someone who frequently compares their appearance to others on Instagram may begin to feel dissatisfied with their own looks, even if those looks are completely normal and healthy. Similarly, comparing one's career path to someone else's success can cause unnecessary stress, self-doubt, and a diminished sense of achievement, even if the individual is progressing at their own pace.

The negative consequences of comparison can extend to mental health issues like anxiety and depression. When self-worth becomes overly dependent on how we measure up to others, we create a fragile foundation for our emotional well-being. In the absence of external validation or recognition, we may feel worthless or unimportant. The fear of not being good enough can lead to imposter syndrome, where individuals believe that they do not deserve their accomplishments, further diminishing their confidence and mental stability.

However, comparison doesn't always have to be harmful. Upward comparison, where we look to those we admire for inspiration or motivation, can be beneficial if it encourages growth.

Yet, the key lies in maintaining a balanced perspective and recognizing that everyone's journey is unique. It's important to remind ourselves that what is shared online often represents only the best, most polished moments of people's lives, and that everyone faces challenges and setbacks that are not visible in the public sphere.

The way comparison affects our self-worth is deeply tied to how we perceive ourselves in relation to others, particularly in the context of social media. Constantly comparing ourselves to curated, idealized versions of other people's lives can lead to diminished self-esteem, dissatisfaction, and mental health struggles. To foster a healthier sense of self-worth, it's essential to practice self-compassion, focus on personal growth, and recognize that our value is not determined by external comparisons but by our unique qualities and achievements.

Breaking the Cycle: Strategies for Healthy Self-Perception

Breaking the cycle of negative self-comparison and fostering healthy self-perception is crucial for maintaining mental and emotional well-being, particularly in the digital age where constant exposure to idealized lives on social media can lead to feelings of inadequacy. Strategies to cultivate a positive self-view focus on shifting the way we evaluate ourselves, developing self-compassion, and minimizing harmful external influences. Here are several effective strategies for fostering healthy self-perception.

One of the first steps in breaking the cycle of negative comparison is practicing self-compassion. Often, individuals are their harshest critics, holding themselves to unattainably high standards. Self-compassion involves treating oneself with the same kindness, understanding, and support that one would offer a friend. When we make mistakes or fall short of our expectations, instead of self-blame or judgment, we can acknowledge our imperfections with kindness and learn from them. Practicing self-compassion allows individuals to embrace their flaws without letting them define their worth, fostering a healthier self-image.

Another important strategy is challenging perfectionism. Perfectionism is closely tied to negative self-comparison, as individuals set unrealistic standards for themselves based on what they see online or in others. Recognizing that perfection is unattainable and that mistakes are a natural part of life can free individuals from the burden of constantly comparing themselves to an idealized version of success or beauty. By accepting that imperfection is part of the human experience, individuals can foster a healthier sense of self and reduce the pressure they place on themselves.

Limiting social media exposure is a practical way to break the cycle of comparison. Social media often presents curated, filtered images of others' lives, which are typically far removed from reality. Taking time to unfollow or mute accounts that make you feel inadequate or trigger comparison can help create a more balanced digital environment. Instead, follow accounts that inspire and uplift you—whether those accounts focus on personal growth, positive body image, or creative inspiration. Reducing exposure to idealized versions of other people's lives gives individuals more space to focus on their own unique journey without feeling pressured by the need to compete.

Fostering gratitude is another powerful tool for building healthy self-perception. Practicing gratitude helps individuals shift their focus from what they lack or compare unfavorably with, to what they already have. Regularly reflecting on the positive aspects of life, including personal strengths, accomplishments, and relationships, helps to shift the narrative from one of lack to one of abundance. Gratitude nurtures a positive mindset, encouraging individuals to appreciate their own journey and growth rather than constantly comparing it to others.

Another key strategy for healthy self-perception is celebrating small wins and acknowledging personal progress. Often, people focus on long-term goals and fail to recognize the value of small steps along the way. Taking time to celebrate incremental successes, whether it's completing a task, learning something new, or improving in a skill, reinforces a positive view of oneself. Recognizing and appreciating personal achievements—no matter how small—encourages feelings of accomplishment and builds confidence.

Lastly, seeking support from others can be vital in breaking the cycle of comparison. Engaging in open, honest conversations with friends, family, or a therapist can provide perspective and reassurance. Talking about struggles and learning from others' experiences helps individuals understand that they are not alone in their feelings of inadequacy and that self-worth does not depend on comparing oneself to others.

Breaking the cycle of negative comparison and cultivating a healthy self-perception requires intention and practice. By practicing self-compassion, challenging perfectionism, limiting exposure to unrealistic portrayals of life, fostering gratitude, celebrating personal achievements, and seeking support, individuals can build a healthier and more balanced sense of self. These strategies help to reduce the impact of external comparisons and allow individuals to embrace their uniqueness, fostering a more fulfilling and positive self-view.

Chapter 9
The Digital Divide: Mental Health in the Age of Inequality

In the digital age, technology has the potential to bring about transformative changes in access to information, education, healthcare, and social connection. However, the benefits of digital advancements are not universally accessible, and the growing reliance on technology has revealed a significant digital divide. This divide is not only about access to devices and the internet but also about how disparities in access to technology contribute to mental health inequality. Those who lack access to digital tools are more likely to experience disadvantages in both mental and physical health, exacerbating existing social and economic inequalities.

The relationship between access to technology and mental health is complex. For individuals in lower socioeconomic groups, the lack of access to technology can limit opportunities for social connection, employment, and mental health support. Meanwhile, those with better access are often better equipped to utilize technology to support their mental health through online therapy, social connections, and educational resources. This gap creates a disparity in digital wellness, with a growing number of individuals left behind in a world that increasingly relies on technology for support and connection.

This chapter will explore how access to technology influences mental health disparities, particularly focusing on how socioeconomic status can significantly affect an individual's ability to maintain digital wellness. We will examine the implications of the digital divide on mental health, highlighting the challenges faced by underserved communities. Additionally, we will discuss solutions and strategies to bridge the gap, including policies and initiatives aimed at ensuring that mental health resources are equally accessible to all, regardless of their socioeconomic background. By addressing these issues, we can begin to promote mental health equity in a world increasingly shaped by technology.

Access to Technology and Mental Health Disparities

Access to technology plays a crucial role in shaping an individual's mental health, influencing how people interact with the world, seek support, and engage in activities that promote well-being. However, the digital divide—the gap between those with access to modern technology and those without—has created significant disparities in mental health outcomes. This divide is especially pronounced among marginalized communities, where socioeconomic factors and limited access to digital tools further exacerbate existing mental health disparities.

For individuals with limited access to technology, the barriers to receiving adequate mental health support are substantial. Online therapy, mental health apps, educational resources, and virtual support groups are increasingly becoming primary sources of help for many people. However, those without reliable access to the internet, smartphones, or computers are excluded from these vital services. This lack of access can prevent individuals from seeking out necessary mental health support, leaving them more vulnerable to untreated mental health issues such as anxiety, depression, and stress. In rural or economically disadvantaged areas, where access to healthcare providers may also be limited, technology is one of the few lifelines to mental health services. Without access to these tools, many individuals are left without sufficient resources to address their mental health needs.

Moreover, access to technology can impact social connection, which is a critical factor in mental well-being. Social isolation has been linked to higher rates of depression and anxiety, and for many, the internet provides an essential platform to maintain relationships, engage in communities, and combat feelings of loneliness. Those with restricted access to technology may struggle to stay connected with friends and family, exacerbating feelings of isolation and contributing to mental health decline. Social media platforms, when used mindfully, can help build social support networks, but for those without access, this form of connection is entirely out of reach.

Furthermore, socioeconomic status is a key determinant of access to technology, and as a result, it plays a significant role in mental health disparities. Low-income individuals are less likely to own personal devices such as smartphones, tablets, or laptops, and they may also face financial barriers that prevent them from accessing high-speed internet. These gaps in access create a cycle where disadvantaged individuals are not only excluded from technological advancements but also lack the resources to engage in activities that can improve their mental health, such as online learning, self-care apps, or fitness programs. For individuals in poverty or facing economic hardship, mental health often becomes a secondary concern behind more immediate challenges like financial stability, housing, and food security.

The mental health disparities created by unequal access to technology extend beyond individuals to entire communities. Marginalized populations—including those in rural areas, communities of color, and low-income families—are disproportionately affected by the digital divide. This inequity in access is compounded by systemic issues in healthcare, education, and social services, which often leave these communities with fewer resources to address mental health needs. The lack of technological access reinforces a cycle of inequality, where the most vulnerable populations face increased barriers to care and support.

The digital divide has a significant impact on mental health disparities, as access to technology plays a crucial role in both the availability and accessibility of mental health resources. Without reliable access to digital tools, many individuals are left behind, unable to fully benefit from the mental health support and services that technology provides. Bridging this gap is essential for ensuring that all individuals, regardless of their socioeconomic background, have the opportunity to achieve better mental health outcomes.

How Socioeconomic Status Affects Digital Wellness

Socioeconomic status (SES) plays a significant role in determining an individual's access to resources, including technology, which in turn affects their digital wellness. Digital wellness refers to the healthy use of technology, including how we manage our digital interactions, balance screen time, and leverage technology for personal well-being. For individuals in lower socioeconomic brackets, the challenges related to digital wellness are compounded by a lack of access to devices, high-speed internet, and digital resources that are increasingly integral to maintaining mental and emotional well-being in today's society.

One of the most significant ways SES impacts digital wellness is through access to technology. People in lower-income households may not have access to personal computers, smartphones, or reliable internet connections, which limits their ability to engage in essential online activities. Digital mental health resources, such as therapy apps, support groups, and educational materials, are increasingly being delivered through online platforms. However, individuals in lower SES brackets may be unable to afford the necessary technology to access these resources. This lack of access creates a barrier to important services that can help manage stress, anxiety, and other mental health challenges, further perpetuating disparities in mental health care.

Furthermore, the absence of reliable internet or devices can hinder education and career opportunities, which directly impacts well-being. In today's world, digital literacy and access to technology are essential for academic and professional success. Students from low-income families may struggle to complete assignments, participate in online learning, or access valuable information due to limited access to devices or high-speed internet. This creates an environment where individuals are already at a disadvantage, making them more vulnerable to stress, frustration, and feelings of inadequacy, all of which affect their digital wellness.

Digital stress is another area where socioeconomic status plays a critical role. Those with limited access to technology often face the stress of trying to make do with outdated or subpar devices. Additionally, digital overload can disproportionately affect individuals in lower SES communities, where the need to constantly be "on" and available through digital platforms (for work, school, or social reasons) can create added pressure. For those in lower-income brackets, who may already be juggling multiple jobs or coping with financial instability, managing digital stress can become overwhelming. The inability to disconnect from work or family obligations due to constant digital connectivity can contribute to burnout and mental health struggles.

Moreover, social isolation can also affect digital wellness in lower SES communities. Social media and other online platforms are often used to maintain connections and combat loneliness, especially for individuals who are geographically or socially isolated. However, those without access to these platforms due to financial constraints may experience increased social isolation, leading to feelings of loneliness, anxiety, and depression. Conversely, excessive use of social media in an attempt to connect with others or escape personal challenges can contribute to negative mental health outcomes. Lower SES groups may also be more susceptible to harmful online behaviors, such as cyberbullying, due to the lack of digital literacy and support systems to navigate online spaces safely.

Socioeconomic status has a profound impact on digital wellness, shaping both access to technology and how individuals engage with it. Those in lower income brackets often face barriers that limit their ability to benefit from the positive aspects of technology, such as mental health resources, educational opportunities, and social connection. Bridging this digital divide requires policy changes that prioritize access to technology, digital literacy programs, and mental health support for underserved communities.

Bridging the Gap: Solutions for Mental Health Equity

Bridging the gap in mental health equity is essential to ensuring that all individuals, regardless of their socioeconomic status, geographic location, or digital access, have equal opportunities to achieve mental wellness. The disparity in access to mental health resources has been exacerbated by socioeconomic factors, such as income inequality, lack of access to technology, and limited availability of care in certain communities. To achieve mental health equity, it is vital to focus on both systemic changes and targeted interventions that address these gaps.

One of the most crucial steps in bridging the mental health equity gap is improving access to affordable mental health care. In many underserved communities, there is a shortage of mental health professionals and services, making it difficult for individuals to receive the care they need. Increasing funding for mental health services in low-income areas and rural communities is essential. This can include funding for public health programs that offer free or low-cost therapy, counseling, and support services. Expanding telehealth services and digital mental health platforms is another way to provide mental health resources in areas where in-person care is not readily available. These platforms can bridge the gap by offering remote therapy, mental health apps, and online support groups to individuals who might otherwise be excluded from care due to geographical or financial barriers.

Another vital solution is enhancing digital literacy in underserved communities. Many individuals in lower socioeconomic brackets struggle with digital literacy, which makes it difficult for them to access online mental health resources or navigate the digital world safely. Providing digital literacy education can empower these individuals to take advantage of the many online resources available for mental wellness, from meditation apps to virtual counseling services. Schools, community centers, and local organizations can play a significant role in offering these educational programs to ensure that all people have the skills needed to thrive in a technology-driven world.

To further promote mental health equity, culturally competent care is essential. Mental health professionals must be trained to understand the cultural contexts and unique challenges faced by individuals from diverse backgrounds, including those from different racial, ethnic, and socioeconomic groups. Providing mental health care that is sensitive to cultural differences can help ensure that all individuals feel understood and supported in their mental health journeys. Incorporating culturally relevant therapy techniques and addressing the specific needs of marginalized populations can make a significant difference in promoting engagement and improving outcomes.

Community-based initiatives can also help reduce disparities in mental health. By creating local support networks, offering community-based mental health programs, and providing peer support, we can foster an environment where individuals feel empowered to seek help. Community mental health programs that focus on building trust and providing support in a familiar, non-judgmental environment can encourage individuals to access care without fear of stigma or discrimination.

Lastly, policy reforms are necessary to address systemic inequalities that contribute to mental health disparities. Advocating for mental health care to be included in universal health coverage, ensuring that mental health is treated with the same urgency and importance as physical health, and creating policies that protect vulnerable populations from discrimination in accessing care are critical steps toward achieving mental health equity.

Bridging the gap in mental health equity requires a multifaceted approach that includes improving access to care, enhancing digital literacy, providing culturally competent services, building community support, and advocating for policy changes. By addressing the systemic barriers that contribute to mental health disparities, we can create a more inclusive and equitable mental health system that supports the well-being of all individuals, regardless of their background or circumstances.

Chapter 10
Children, Teens, and Screen Time

As digital technology becomes increasingly embedded in daily life, children and teenagers are spending more time on screens than ever before. Social media, in particular, has become a significant part of adolescent culture, influencing how young people interact with the world around them. While the internet and digital devices offer educational opportunities, creativity, and social connection, excessive screen time can also have detrimental effects on adolescent development. The impact of social media on self-esteem, social skills, and emotional well-being is a growing concern, as teens are exposed to a constant stream of idealized images, social comparisons, and online pressures.

Parents and caregivers face the challenge of navigating their children's screen time in a digital landscape that is ever-changing. Finding the right balance between encouraging the positive aspects of technology and setting boundaries to protect their mental and emotional health is crucial. This requires a proactive approach that includes clear rules, monitoring, and engaging with children in conversations about healthy screen habits.

As young people are still developing emotionally, socially, and cognitively, their relationship with technology can significantly influence their self-image, social interactions, and overall well-being. Thus, fostering healthy digital habits and ensuring that children have a balanced approach to screen time is more important than ever. In this chapter, we will explore the impact of social media on adolescent development, focusing on how it influences self-esteem, body image, and social interactions. Additionally, we will discuss the role of parents in managing screen time, offering strategies for setting effective boundaries and teaching kids how to engage with digital media responsibly. By fostering a healthy relationship with technology, we can ensure that children and teens thrive in the digital age while maintaining their mental and emotional health.

The Impact of Social Media on Adolescent Development

Social media has become a central part of adolescent life, significantly influencing their development, self-esteem, and mental health. While social media platforms offer opportunities for connection, self-expression, and entertainment, they also pose unique challenges for young people as they navigate the complexities of growing up in the digital age. The impact of social media on adolescent development can be both positive and negative, with potential long-term consequences on emotional well-being, identity formation, and social behavior.

One of the most notable impacts of social media on adolescents is its effect on self-esteem and body image. Platforms like Instagram and TikTok, which emphasize visual content, can encourage young people to compare themselves to the highly curated, often idealized images they see online. These comparisons can foster feelings of inadequacy and dissatisfaction with one's body, especially when young people view influencers or celebrities who appear to lead "perfect" lives. Research has shown that social comparison on social media is linked to body dysmorphia, low self-esteem, and eating disorders. For adolescents who are still developing their sense of identity, these comparisons can have a lasting impact on how they perceive themselves and their value.

Furthermore, the constant need for validation on social media platforms can exacerbate these issues. Teenagers are particularly susceptible to external approval, and the "likes," comments, and shares they receive on posts can become a measure of their worth. The pursuit of social validation can drive young people to carefully curate their online personas, often showing only the best and most glamorous aspects of their lives while hiding struggles or vulnerabilities. This can create a distorted sense of reality, leading adolescents to believe that their lives must align with the perfection they see online. Over time, this need for validation can lead to anxiety and depression when the feedback doesn't meet expectations.

Social media also has a significant impact on social development. While platforms can foster connections and friendships, they can also facilitate social isolation. Adolescents who spend excessive time on social media may withdraw from face-to-face interactions, which are essential for developing interpersonal skills, emotional intelligence, and empathy. Additionally, the nature of online interactions can often be superficial, lacking the depth and authenticity of in-person communication. This can hinder the development of meaningful relationships, leaving adolescents feeling lonely or disconnected despite having a large online following.

Moreover, cyberbullying has become a pervasive issue in the digital world. Adolescents are particularly vulnerable to online harassment, which can have severe psychological consequences. The anonymity of the internet can embolden bullies, and the 24/7 nature of social media means that victims of cyberbullying often feel trapped in an ongoing cycle of abuse. Studies show that cyberbullying is linked to increased levels of anxiety, depression, and even suicidal ideation in adolescents.

Despite these challenges, social media can also have positive effects on adolescent development. It can provide opportunities for self-expression, creativity, and learning. Social media platforms can connect young people to communities of like-minded individuals, offering support networks that might not be available in their immediate physical environment. For example, teens facing mental health struggles, identity issues, or niche interests may find solace and understanding through online groups and forums. Additionally, social media can be a valuable tool for learning, as educational resources and informative content are widely accessible.

The impact of social media on adolescent development is complex and multifaceted. While it offers opportunities for connection, self-expression, and learning, it also presents significant risks related to self-esteem, body image, social skills, and mental health. Adolescents need guidance and support from parents, educators, and mental health professionals to navigate the digital world in a healthy way. By fostering awareness of the potential negative effects and promoting balanced social media use, we can help adolescents build a positive relationship with technology while prioritizing their emotional and social well-being.

Parental Control and Setting Boundaries

Parental control and setting boundaries are essential components in managing adolescents' screen time and ensuring their digital well-being. As children and teens spend an increasing amount of time online, it's crucial for parents to take an active role in guiding their digital experiences, helping them navigate potential risks while fostering healthy digital habits. Setting clear, consistent boundaries can help mitigate the negative effects of excessive screen time, such as exposure to harmful content, cyberbullying, or social media-induced anxiety, while also encouraging more meaningful offline activities.

One of the first steps in establishing effective parental control is open communication. Parents should have ongoing conversations with their children about their online activities, the content they are accessing, and their experiences on digital platforms. These discussions can help parents understand their child's digital environment and provide an opportunity to establish expectations and rules for screen time. Communication about digital safety, privacy, and respectful online behavior is crucial in fostering a sense of responsibility and awareness about the potential risks associated with online engagement.

Setting time limits is a fundamental aspect of parental control. Excessive screen time has been linked to several negative outcomes, including sleep disturbances, poor academic performance, and physical health issues such as obesity. By establishing daily or weekly limits for recreational screen time, parents can ensure that their children engage in a balanced lifestyle. For instance, limiting the amount of time spent on social media or video games and encouraging alternative activities such as reading, outdoor play, or hobbies can foster a healthier relationship with technology. Tools like screen time tracking apps or built-in parental controls on smartphones, tablets, and computers can help parents monitor and enforce these limits.

Filtering and blocking inappropriate content is another critical aspect of parental control. With the vast amount of content available online, not all of it is suitable for children and teens. Parents should use content filters, web blockers, or child-friendly browsers to limit access to explicit or harmful material. Many devices and apps offer built-in parental controls that allow parents to set age-appropriate content restrictions. This ensures that adolescents are not exposed to inappropriate material, such as violent videos, explicit content, or harmful social media trends.

Social media monitoring is an essential part of setting boundaries for older children and teens who are active on platforms like Instagram, Snapchat, and TikTok. While complete surveillance may not be ideal as children grow older, parents can still stay involved by reviewing privacy settings, tracking friends and followers, and having periodic check-ins about their child's experiences on these platforms. It is also helpful to encourage transparency by setting clear expectations for sharing passwords or being involved in online conversations. While respecting privacy is important, parental involvement in a child's social media activity can help prevent cyberbullying, online predators, and other risks.

Finally, leading by example is one of the most effective ways to set boundaries and model healthy screen time habits. Parents should also be mindful of their own digital behavior, as children tend to mimic their parents' actions. By setting their own boundaries around screen use—such as avoiding excessive phone checking during family time or limiting evening screen time—parents can demonstrate the importance of balancing the digital and real worlds.

Parental control and setting boundaries around screen time are vital for promoting healthy digital habits in children and teens. By engaging in open communication, setting clear limits on screen use, filtering inappropriate content, monitoring social media use, and modeling good behavior, parents can help their children navigate the digital world safely and responsibly. These strategies not only protect children from potential online harms but also encourage a more balanced, mindful approach to technology use that prioritizes emotional, social, and physical well-being.

Teaching Kids Healthy Digital Habits

Teaching kids healthy digital habits is essential for ensuring they develop a positive and balanced relationship with technology. In an increasingly digital world, children and teenagers are exposed to screens from a very young age. Whether it's for entertainment, education, or socializing, technology plays a significant role in their lives. However, without proper guidance, excessive screen time can lead to negative consequences, such as social isolation, poor mental health, and physical issues like poor posture or eye strain. Teaching kids healthy digital habits helps them use technology in a way that enhances their lives while minimizing its potential harms.

One of the first and most important steps in teaching healthy digital habits is modeling balanced screen use. Children learn by observing their parents and caregivers, so it's essential for adults to set a good example. If children see their parents constantly checking their phones or spending excessive time online, they are more likely to mimic those behaviors. Parents can set boundaries for their own screen use, such as designating phone-free times during meals or family activities. Modeling mindful and responsible use of technology is key to teaching kids that screens should complement life, not dominate it.

Setting clear and consistent rules around screen time is another crucial aspect of fostering healthy digital habits. Establishing daily or weekly limits on recreational screen use helps children balance their digital activities with other essential aspects of their lives, such as physical activity, sleep, and face-to-face interactions. For younger children, parents can use screen time management tools, like built-in timers on devices or third-party apps, to enforce these limits. For older children and teens, parents can have ongoing discussions about the importance of time management and allow them to take responsibility for monitoring their screen time.

It's also important to teach kids about digital etiquette and the ethical use of technology. Kids should learn the basics of responsible online behavior, such as treating others with respect, understanding the permanence of online content, and recognizing the potential consequences of sharing personal information. Teaching children about privacy settings, the risks of oversharing, and how to handle inappropriate content or cyberbullying equips them with the skills needed to navigate the online world safely. Encouraging kids to speak up if they feel uncomfortable online and ensuring they know they can turn to trusted adults for guidance is crucial for their emotional safety.

Encouraging offline activities is another essential strategy for promoting healthy digital habits. While technology offers many benefits, it's important to ensure that children engage in offline activities that foster creativity, critical thinking, and physical well-being. Encouraging kids to read, play outside, engage in sports, or pursue hobbies that don't involve screens helps them develop a well-rounded lifestyle. Parents can set aside specific times during the day for these activities, ensuring that they become an integral part of the child's routine.

Finally, teaching digital mindfulness helps children be more intentional about their online behaviors. This involves encouraging kids to reflect on how they feel after using technology. Do they feel happy and energized, or do they feel drained and anxious? Encouraging kids to take regular breaks from screens, practice mindfulness exercises, and avoid excessive multitasking can help them cultivate a balanced approach to technology. This mindfulness helps them recognize when they are becoming overwhelmed or overstimulated by digital content and take steps to reset.

Teaching kids healthy digital habits is about fostering a balanced, intentional relationship with technology. By modeling healthy screen use, setting boundaries, teaching digital etiquette, encouraging offline activities, and promoting digital mindfulness, parents can help their children navigate the digital world safely and responsibly. These habits not only protect children from the negative impacts of excessive screen time but also empower them to use technology in ways that enhance their well-being and personal growth.

Chapter 11
Digital Addiction: Causes, Consequences, and Solutions

In today's technology-driven world, digital addiction has become a growing concern, with an increasing number of people spending excessive amounts of time on digital devices. Whether it's social media, gaming, or constant internet browsing, the overuse of technology is becoming a significant part of daily life, often to the detriment of personal health, relationships, and overall well-being. What starts as casual use can quickly escalate into an addictive pattern, where individuals find themselves unable to control their digital consumption despite the negative impact on their lives.

The addictive nature of technology is fueled by several factors, including the instant gratification provided by notifications, likes, and rewards, which trigger the brain's pleasure centers. The design of many apps, games, and platforms is engineered to keep users engaged for as long as possible, creating a cycle of dependence. Social media platforms, in particular, use algorithms to keep users scrolling, while gaming and entertainment apps use features like achievements, leveling up, and peer comparisons to keep individuals coming back for more.

The consequences of digital addiction are far-reaching, impacting both psychological and physical health. Mentally, digital addiction can lead to issues such as anxiety, depression, and sleep disturbances, as the constant connection to screens disrupts real-life interactions and emotional regulation. Physically, prolonged screen time contributes to eye strain, poor posture, and sedentary lifestyles, which can lead to chronic health issues such as obesity, headaches, and carpal tunnel syndrome.

In this chapter, we will explore the causes of digital addiction, the psychological and physical toll it takes on individuals, and the various treatment approaches available for managing and overcoming digital dependency. Understanding these factors is crucial in addressing the growing concern of digital addiction and finding solutions that can help individuals lead healthier, more balanced lives in an increasingly digital world.

Why Technology is Addictive

Technology is addictive for several reasons, most of which are rooted in the way it interacts with the brain's reward system. Devices and platforms are designed to be engaging, often employing psychological principles that trigger pleasure and reinforcement, which encourages users to continue interacting with them. This interaction with technology often leads to habitual use, where individuals find themselves unable to limit their screen time or break free from the cycle of constant digital engagement.

One of the key reasons technology is addictive is instant gratification. The immediate feedback we receive when using digital platforms—whether it's likes on a post, messages from friends, or rewards in a game—activates the brain's pleasure centers, releasing dopamine, the "feel-good" neurotransmitter. This release of dopamine reinforces the behavior, making it more likely that individuals will return to their devices or social media apps to experience that same sense of reward. Over time, the brain becomes conditioned to seek out these rewarding experiences, leading to a cycle of compulsive use. The variable reward system, which involves random intervals of rewards (such as the unpredictability of receiving likes or messages), also intensifies this effect. The unpredictability of the reward increases the urge to keep checking, as users never know when they might receive the next reward.

Another factor that makes technology addictive is the desire for social connection. Social media platforms, in particular, are designed to keep users engaged by allowing them to connect, share, and interact with others. Humans are inherently social beings, and the need for social interaction is deeply ingrained in our psyche. Digital platforms exploit this by creating a sense of social validation through likes, comments, and shares. The constant pursuit of validation and approval from others can become all-consuming, making users feel compelled to keep engaging with these platforms to maintain their social connections or status.

FOMO (Fear of Missing Out) also plays a significant role in making technology addictive. As users see updates from friends, family, or celebrities, they may feel left out or disconnected from the ongoing conversations or events. This fear of missing out on what's happening in the digital world drives users to check their devices constantly, even when they know they've already seen the latest updates. The need to stay in the loop and remain informed becomes a compulsion, further driving screen time and engagement.

Additionally, the design of technology itself encourages prolonged use. Many apps and websites use endless scrolling, autoplay features, or notifications that pull users back into the platform. These features are designed to make users stay on a platform for longer periods, whether it's watching videos, browsing social media feeds, or engaging in online gaming. The constant availability of new content, combined with the desire for immediate gratification, leads to an unending cycle of engagement.

Finally, personalization also plays a significant role in making technology addictive. Digital platforms use sophisticated algorithms to tailor content to individual preferences, making each user's experience feel unique and relevant. By analyzing user behavior, these platforms deliver content that is more likely to captivate and engage them, creating a sense of personalization that keeps individuals hooked. Whether it's recommended videos on YouTube or curated Instagram feeds, the continuous stream of tailored content ensures that users remain interested, often losing track of time.

Technology is addictive because it taps into fundamental psychological mechanisms—instant gratification, social validation, fear of missing out, and the desire for personalization. The more individuals interact with technology, the more the brain becomes conditioned to seek out these rewards, making it difficult to break free from the cycle of compulsive digital engagement. Understanding these psychological underpinnings is essential for addressing the growing concern of technology addiction and for developing strategies to manage screen time in a healthier, more balanced way.

The Psychological and Physical Toll of Digital Addiction

Digital addiction has significant psychological and physical tolls that can affect nearly every aspect of an individual's well-being. As technology becomes increasingly embedded in daily life, the overuse of digital devices and online platforms is leading to serious consequences, from emotional distress to physical health issues. These effects not only disrupt daily functioning but can also lead to long-term consequences if left unchecked.

Psychologically, the most immediate consequence of digital addiction is the impact on mental health. Constant engagement with screens, especially social media, can lead to heightened anxiety and depression. Social comparison, where individuals compare their lives to the often idealized portrayals of others online, contributes significantly to these feelings. The curated nature of social media creates unrealistic standards of beauty, success, and happiness, which can make individuals feel inadequate or as though they are failing in comparison to others. This contributes to a negative self-image and can lead to low self-esteem.

Additionally, the constant flow of information can lead to information overload, a state in which the brain becomes overwhelmed by excessive digital stimuli. This can impair cognitive function, making it difficult to focus, retain information, or think clearly. As users become accustomed to the fast-paced, immediate feedback provided by digital platforms, they may struggle with attention span and concentration in non-digital environments, leading to difficulties at school, work, or in personal relationships.

The addictive nature of technology also affects emotional regulation. Constant notifications and updates can trigger feelings of urgency and stress, as individuals feel compelled to respond immediately to messages, emails, or social media posts. This creates a heightened state of alertness, which keeps the body in a constant fight-or-flight mode, leading to chronic stress. Over time, this can contribute to more severe mental health conditions, including burnout, insomnia, and post-traumatic stress disorder (PTSD), especially in individuals who are consistently overwhelmed by the demands of digital communication.

Physically, digital addiction has been linked to a variety of health problems. Prolonged screen time, particularly from mobile devices and computers, contributes to eye strain, headaches, and sleep disturbances. The blue light emitted by screens interferes with the body's production of melatonin, the hormone responsible for regulating sleep, leading to difficulties falling asleep or maintaining quality sleep. This disruption in sleep cycles can result in chronic fatigue, irritability, and cognitive dysfunction, further exacerbating the psychological toll.

Another physical consequence is related to sedentary behavior. Digital addiction often leads to prolonged sitting, whether watching TV, playing video games, or using social media. This lack of physical activity increases the risk of obesity, heart disease, and other chronic health conditions. The extended use of digital devices also contributes to poor posture, which can result in neck pain, back pain, and other musculoskeletal issues. These physical health issues, compounded by the psychological stress of digital addiction, can further reduce an individual's quality of life.

The impact of digital addiction on both mental and physical health is substantial, and without intervention, these effects can become ingrained, leading to long-term difficulties. It is essential to take proactive steps to limit screen time, practice digital mindfulness, and engage in offline activities to restore balance and protect overall health. Strategies such as regular breaks from screens, setting boundaries around technology use, and fostering healthy offline habits can significantly reduce the psychological and physical toll of digital addiction, promoting a more balanced and healthier lifestyle.

Treatment Approaches for Digital Dependency

Treatment approaches for digital dependency are becoming increasingly essential as more individuals struggle with the psychological, emotional, and physical toll of excessive screen time and digital engagement. While digital technology offers numerous benefits, its overuse can lead to serious consequences, such as anxiety, depression, social isolation, and physical health issues. Fortunately, various strategies and therapeutic approaches can help individuals reduce their dependency on digital devices and regain control of their lives.

One of the most effective approaches for treating digital dependency is cognitive-behavioral therapy (CBT). CBT is a well-established therapeutic technique that helps individuals identify and change negative thought patterns and behaviors. In the case of digital addiction, CBT can assist individuals in recognizing the harmful thoughts and emotional responses that drive excessive screen use. By learning to replace these thoughts with healthier, more balanced coping strategies, individuals can begin to reduce their screen time and engage in more fulfilling offline activities. CBT also helps people develop better time management skills, enabling them to set boundaries and prioritize activities that support their mental and physical well-being.

Another important treatment approach is digital detox. A digital detox involves intentionally disconnecting from digital devices for a specified period of time to break the cycle of dependency. This approach can be done gradually, by reducing screen time incrementally, or more radically by taking a complete break from screens for a set period, such as a weekend or weeklong retreat. The goal of a digital detox is to allow individuals to reset their relationship with technology, reduce stress, and regain a sense of balance. During this time, individuals are encouraged to engage in activities that foster social connection, physical activity, and creativity, such as spending time outdoors, reading, or pursuing hobbies that don't involve screens.

Mindfulness practices are also an effective treatment for digital dependency. Mindfulness involves being fully present in the moment without judgment, which can help individuals become more aware of their digital habits and the emotional impact of excessive screen use. Practicing mindfulness techniques, such as deep breathing, meditation, and body scans, allows individuals to reconnect with themselves and reduce the urge to constantly check their devices. Mindfulness encourages individuals to observe their thoughts and feelings surrounding technology use, helping them create healthier habits and reduce stress associated with digital engagement.

For those struggling with more severe forms of digital addiction, professional counseling or therapy may be necessary.

Mental health professionals who specialize in addiction treatment can work with individuals to explore the underlying causes of their dependency, such as emotional distress, social isolation, or low self-esteem. Counseling provides a safe space for individuals to process their emotions, develop coping strategies, and receive support in overcoming their addiction. In some cases, group therapy or support groups, such as those focused on internet addiction or technology dependence, can provide additional support and help individuals connect with others facing similar challenges.

Finally, setting boundaries and establishing healthy digital habits are crucial steps in managing digital dependency. Parents, educators, and employers can play an important role in encouraging healthy screen time practices. For children and teens, setting time limits on recreational device use, monitoring screen activities, and ensuring that devices are put away during family time or before bedtime can help reduce screen addiction. For adults, creating screen-free zones (e.g., bedrooms or dining areas), setting designated times for checking email or social media, and using apps that track and limit screen time can all contribute to a healthier digital lifestyle.

Treatment for digital dependency requires a multifaceted approach, including therapies such as cognitive-behavioral therapy, digital detoxes, mindfulness practices, professional counseling, and the establishment of boundaries. By combining these strategies, individuals can break free from digital addiction, regain balance, and improve their overall mental and physical well-being. Reducing screen time is essential for fostering healthier relationships with technology and creating a more fulfilling, present life.

Chapter 12
Digital Addiction: Causes, Consequences, and Solutions

In the digital age, where technology permeates nearly every aspect of daily life, creating a healthy digital environment is essential for maintaining mental well-being and balance. While technology offers countless benefits, including convenience, connectivity, and access to information, it can also lead to overwhelming stress, digital burnout, and unhealthy habits if not used mindfully. The key to a healthy relationship with technology lies in how we engage with it—setting boundaries, designing a mindful digital routine, and building a supportive community are crucial steps in ensuring that technology enhances rather than detracts from our lives.

Setting boundaries is an important aspect of creating a healthy digital environment. Without limits, digital devices can become all-consuming, leading to feelings of anxiety, social isolation, and exhaustion. Self-regulation is essential in managing how we use technology, allowing us to prioritize meaningful activities, focus on offline relationships, and ensure that our digital interactions align with our values and goals.

In addition to setting boundaries, designing a mindful digital routine can help us establish healthy habits and create a sense of structure. A mindful digital routine involves intentional use of technology that supports personal growth, reduces stress, and fosters productivity. This can include scheduling time for digital detoxes, incorporating mindfulness practices, and setting aside time for non-digital activities such as exercise, hobbies, or quality time with loved ones.

Lastly, building a supportive digital community is vital for cultivating a positive online environment. Engaging with like-minded individuals and communities that promote healthy, respectful communication and personal development can enhance the digital experience. By surrounding ourselves with people who encourage growth, well-being, and positive digital habits, we can foster a healthier online environment that promotes connection and support.

We will explore the importance of setting digital boundaries, creating a mindful routine, and building a supportive community to maintain a healthy and fulfilling relationship with technology. These strategies will help individuals engage with the digital world in a way that benefits both their mental and emotional well-being.

Setting Boundaries: The Role of Self-Regulation

Setting boundaries and practicing self-regulation are fundamental to maintaining a healthy relationship with technology in today's digital age. The constant presence of screens, social media, and notifications has made it increasingly difficult to disconnect and prioritize well-being. Without clear boundaries, technology can quickly overwhelm our daily lives, leading to stress, burnout, and disrupted personal relationships. The role of self-regulation in setting these boundaries is essential, as it enables individuals to regain control over their technology use and create a balanced, intentional digital environment.

Self-regulation refers to the ability to manage one's behavior, emotions, and thoughts in the face of external demands, such as the constant pull of digital devices. In the context of digital consumption, self-regulation involves setting conscious limits on screen time, prioritizing offline activities, and making intentional decisions about how and when to engage with technology. The first step in practicing self-regulation is becoming aware of technology usage patterns. Many individuals are unaware of just how much time they spend on their devices or how often they check their phones. Tracking screen time through built-in apps on smartphones or using third-party apps can provide valuable insights into one's habits and help identify areas where technology use can be reduced.

Setting clear, manageable boundaries for screen time is one of the most effective self-regulation strategies. This can include limiting the number of hours spent on social media, setting specific times for checking emails or news, or scheduling phone-free periods during meals or before bed. By consciously choosing when to engage with technology, individuals can reduce the risk of mindless scrolling or excessive device use, which can lead to negative emotional or psychological effects. For example, enforcing a rule of no screens for an hour before sleep can significantly improve sleep quality and overall well-being, as it helps regulate the body's natural sleep cycles and reduces overstimulation.

Creating tech-free zones within the home is another useful self-regulation strategy. By designating areas such as the dining room or bedroom as screen-free zones, individuals can ensure that these spaces are reserved for in-person interactions, relaxation, or sleep. These boundaries help create a healthier work-life balance, as technology is no longer allowed to invade personal and family spaces. Additionally, setting boundaries around work-related technology use, such as turning off work emails during weekends or vacations, allows individuals to fully disconnect and recharge.

In addition to time-based boundaries, emotional self-regulation is an essential part of managing technology use. For instance, setting limits on emotionally charged content, such as following news or social media accounts that may trigger negative feelings, helps prevent unnecessary stress and anxiety. Practicing mindfulness when using technology—by pausing to check in with one's emotions or taking a deep breath before responding to a notification—can help individuals maintain a sense of control over their reactions and avoid impulsive or reactive behavior.

Ultimately, the ability to self-regulate is what empowers individuals to create a balanced digital life. By setting boundaries around screen time, emotional responses, and device use, individuals can ensure that technology supports, rather than hinders, their personal well-being. Self-regulation fosters intentional engagement with digital content, which promotes healthier mental, emotional, and physical outcomes. With consistent practice, setting boundaries through self-regulation becomes a powerful tool for reclaiming control over our relationship with technology and creating a healthier, more mindful digital environment.

How to Design a Mindful Digital Routine

Designing a mindful digital routine is essential for fostering a balanced and healthy relationship with technology. With the constant availability of screens and digital content, it's easy to become overwhelmed, distracted, or consumed by technology. A mindful digital routine encourages intentional engagement with devices, ensuring that technology enhances rather than detracts from our daily lives. By establishing structured boundaries, integrating mindfulness practices, and prioritizing meaningful activities, individuals can regain control over their digital habits and reduce the stress associated with digital overload.

The first step in designing a mindful digital routine is to establish clear goals and priorities for your technology use. Before diving into digital activities, consider what you want to achieve or experience online. Is it staying connected with loved ones? Gaining new knowledge through educational content? Relaxing through entertainment or mindfulness apps? By defining your purpose for digital engagement, you can focus on meaningful interactions rather than mindlessly scrolling or jumping from one app to another. Setting these clear intentions helps prevent unnecessary distractions and enhances productivity.

Next, set specific time limits for digital use. Without boundaries, it's easy to get caught in the endless loop of notifications, emails, or social media feeds. Time-blocking can be a highly effective method for structuring digital engagement. For example, designate 30 minutes in the morning for checking emails, 20 minutes for social media updates, and 1 hour in the evening for leisure activities like watching TV or reading articles. Once these time slots are used up, engage in a tech-free activity. This method not only curtails excessive screen time but also helps maintain balance by ensuring that online interactions don't interfere with offline activities, such as family time, exercise, or personal hobbies.

Incorporate regular digital detoxes into your routine to give yourself time to recharge and reset. A digital detox can range from small practices, like turning off notifications for a few hours, to larger breaks, such as designating one day a week to be screen-free. These periods of disconnection are crucial for reducing digital stress and fostering greater focus and mindfulness. Use this time to engage in offline activities, such as taking a walk, practicing a hobby, or meditating, which allows you to reconnect with the present moment.

Curate the content you consume mindfully. In the age of information overload, it's essential to be selective about the digital content you engage with. Avoid overwhelming yourself with unnecessary news, negative social media feeds, or irrelevant advertisements. Follow accounts, join groups, and subscribe to content that brings value, positivity, or learning to your life. Curating your digital environment ensures that the content you consume supports your mental health and personal goals rather than contributing to stress or anxiety.

Additionally, practice mindfulness while engaging with technology. This involves being fully present in whatever digital activity you're doing, whether it's responding to an email, watching a video, or scrolling through social media. Instead of mindlessly going through your feed or rushing through tasks, pause and check in with yourself. Are you focused and engaged? How does this activity make you feel? Taking moments to reflect and breathe while using technology can help prevent stress and increase your awareness of how digital activities impact your emotions.

Finally, set tech-free zones in your home or workspace to maintain a balance between online and offline life. Designate certain areas for relaxation, eating, or sleeping that are free from digital devices. This helps create a clear boundary between work or digital consumption and personal, offline time. When you remove screens from spaces where you need to rest or focus, it promotes healthier sleep habits and allows for deeper relaxation and connection with others.

Designing a mindful digital routine is about creating structure, intentionality, and balance in your technology use. By setting goals, limiting screen time, curating content, incorporating regular breaks, and practicing mindfulness, you can manage your digital habits in a way that supports your well-being. This approach reduces stress, enhances focus, and fosters a more positive, balanced relationship with technology. With a mindful digital routine, technology becomes a tool for growth and productivity rather than a source of overwhelm or distraction.

Building a Supportive Digital Community

Building a supportive digital community is an essential step in fostering a healthy relationship with technology and ensuring that our online interactions contribute to our well-being. In the digital age, social media and online platforms have become major spaces for connection, but not all online communities are positive or supportive. For individuals seeking a safe and enriching environment online, it's crucial to actively seek out and build digital communities that are grounded in respect, encouragement, and mutual growth. A supportive digital community offers a space where individuals can share experiences, seek advice, and build meaningful connections without fear of judgment, toxicity, or negativity.

The first step in building a supportive digital community is to identify your values and the kind of environment you want to be part of. Whether you're looking for support related to mental health, fitness, hobbies, parenting, or professional growth, it's important to choose communities that align with your personal values. Start by following accounts or joining online groups that promote positivity, inclusivity, and open-mindedness. Avoid spaces that encourage toxic behavior, comparison, or hostility. Your digital community should be a place where you feel safe to express yourself, ask questions, and seek advice.

Next, engage authentically in the communities you join. Building a supportive network goes beyond just being a passive observer. Actively participate by sharing your experiences, offering help to others, and contributing to discussions in a meaningful way. This not only enriches the community but also strengthens your connections within it. A supportive community thrives when its members genuinely care for one another, and this can only happen when individuals are open, honest, and willing to engage authentically.

Another important aspect of creating a supportive digital environment is setting healthy boundaries. While it's essential to engage with others, it's also crucial to know when to step back and protect your mental health. If certain conversations or interactions become overwhelming or stressful, take a break or unfollow accounts that are no longer serving you in a positive way. A supportive community respects personal boundaries and understands that each member's emotional well-being is important. Ensure that the groups or individuals you engage with respect these boundaries and encourage healthy interactions.

Promoting mutual support and empathy is another key component of building a supportive digital community. Foster an environment where individuals uplift one another, celebrate achievements, and provide encouragement during challenging times. This can be done by acknowledging others' milestones, offering words of encouragement, and showing empathy when someone shares a difficult experience. A community based on mutual support not only provides emotional comfort but also strengthens relationships between members, creating a sense of belonging and trust.

Finally, moderation and guidelines are essential in maintaining the integrity of a supportive community. As communities grow, it becomes more challenging to ensure that conversations stay respectful and that harmful behavior is addressed. Establishing clear guidelines for respectful conduct and ensuring that moderators are active in upholding these standards is essential to keeping the community safe. Communities should have systems in place to report harassment or inappropriate behavior, ensuring that members feel protected and valued.